D0457267

living
without
plastic

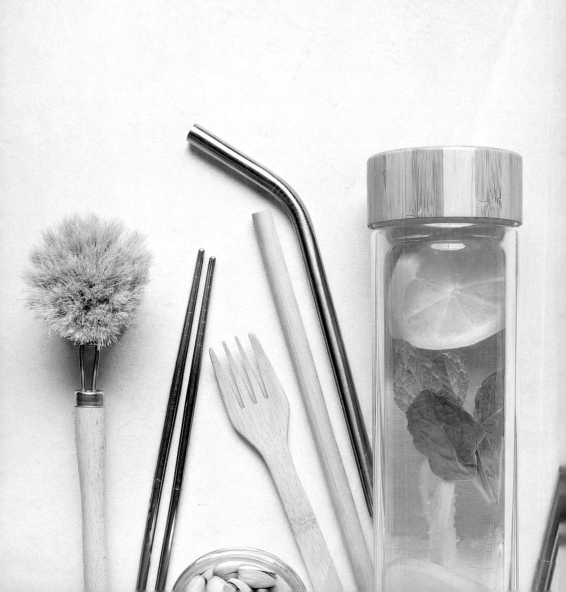

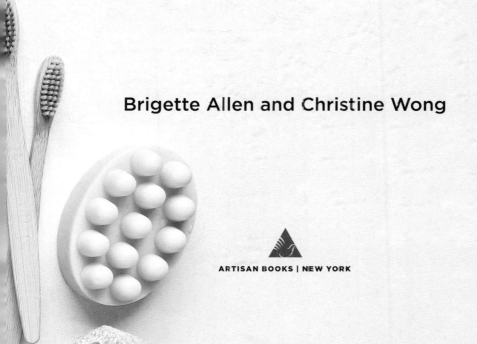

living without plastic

More than 100 Easy Swaps for Home,
Travel, Dining, Holidays, and Beyond

Brigette Allen and Christine Wong

ARTISAN BOOKS | NEW YORK

Copyright © 2020 by Plastic Oceans International and Christine Wong
Photography credits can be found on page 251.

All rights reserved. No portion of this book may be reproduced—mechanically, electronically, or by any other means, including photocopying—without written permission of the publisher.

Library of Congress Cataloging-in-Publication Data

Names: Allen, Brigette, author. | Wong, Christine, 1968- author.
Title: Living without plastic : more than 100 easy swaps for home, travel, dining, holidays, and beyond / Brigette Allen and Christine Wong.
Description: New York, NY : Artisan, a division of Workman Publishing Co., Inc., [2020] | Includes index.
Identifiers: LCCN 2020015896 | ISBN 9781579659400 (hardcover)
Subjects: LCSH: Plastics—Environmental aspects. | Environmental protection—Citizen participation. | Waste minimization. | Sustainable living.
Classification: LCC TD798 .A45 2020 | DDC 640.28/6—dc23
LC record available at https://lccn.loc.gov/2020015896

ISBN 978-1-57965-940-0

Design by Suet Chong
Front cover photograph: Christine Wong
Back cover photograph: Sentelia/Shutterstock
Cover design: Suet Chong

Artisan books are available at special discounts when purchased in bulk for premiums and sales promotions as well as for fund-raising or educational use. Special editions or book excerpts also can be created to specification. For details, contact the Special Sales Director at the address below, or send an e-mail to specialmarkets@workman.com.

For speaking engagements, contact speakersbureau@workman.com.

Published by Artisan
A division of Workman Publishing Co., Inc.
225 Varick Street
New York, NY 10014-4381
artisanbooks.com

Artisan is a registered trademark of Workman Publishing Co., Inc.

Published simultaneously in Canada by Thomas Allen & Son, Limited

Printed in China

First printing, October 2020

10 9 8 7 6 5 4 3 2 1

Disclaimer
This publication contains the opinions and ideas of its authors. It is intended to provide helpful and informative material on the subjects addressed in the publication. It is sold with the understanding that the authors and the publisher are not engaged in rendering medical, health, or any other kind of services in the book. The reader should consult his or her medical, health, or other competent professional before adopting any of the suggestions in this book or drawing any inferences from it.

CONTENTS

Foreword by Julie Andersen   7

Introduction   9

ONE   **At Home**   23

TWO   **Food and Drink**   83

THREE   **Health and Beauty**   125

FOUR   **On the Go**   161

FIVE   **Special Occasions**   187

30-Day Plastic Detox Plan   221

Resources   233
Sources   243
Acknowledgments   250
Photo Credits   251
Index   252

FOREWORD

Plastic is an incredible invention that has helped democratize the world. Plastics have improved modern life, from food safety and access to goods and transportation, to medical sanitation and more.

Unfortunately, the ubiquity of plastic demonstrates that we do not have just a simple plastic habit, but rather a serious relationship with it. Versatile, lightweight, durable and affordable, plastic is a difficult material to replace. And yet despite the growing evidence of the negative impacts of plastic on the environment, animal health, and even human health, many people find it difficult to end this very convenient relationship. We are faced with the dilemma of trying to find a balance between human convenience and environmental impact.

Fortunately, this type of dilemma is not new. Our relationship to our environment—whether personal or physical—develops for a reason. As we learn new information and gain new perspectives, we grow and change.

Now more than ever—for the good of our health, our families and friends, and our planet—we need to change our relationship with plastic.

"Sometimes good things fall apart so better things can fall together."
                                                    —Marilyn Monroe

Living Without Plastic demonstrates how new perspectives come together to help us reduce our use of plastic. Rethinking plastic can start with a single change, and the solutions found in this book show the wonderful opportunities to move forward with plastic alternatives. The accompanying facts provide new insight on the large reach of the harm caused by plastic and help support our choice to make changes.

Plastic is integrated into every aspect of our lives. It can feel like a monumental task to change the way you interact with so many of your daily items, whether it's your cup of coffee or the spoon you use to stir it. However, Christine and Brigette have left no stone unturned and fully delve into sourcing various alternatives and solutions, presenting the options in a way that allows us to select one small swap or all of them, in a way that best fits our lives.

This book represents the power we have as individuals and how, together, our actions create social change—a change away from plastic pollution and toward a better you and a better planet.

Julie Andersen
Plastic Oceans International

INTRODUCTION

It would be difficult to get through your day without encountering plastic. It is in virtually everything we use—electronics, cars, furniture, building materials, clothes, shoes, medical equipment, and kitchen appliances. It is also prevalent with single-use packaging like water bottles and shopping bags that are used for only a short period of time and then discarded. While it is convenient and inexpensive, plastic does not biodegrade, so it accumulates in landfills and in our environment. This book explores the most common plastic items we use on a daily basis in our homes and offices and on the go so you can identify where you use plastic most in your life and adopt simple solutions to reduce your usage. Each swap or adjustment we implement will make a difference.

History

The earliest plastic was made from plant cellulose, not petroleum, and was created in the late 1800s as a solution to replace materials acquired inhumanely, such as ivory and tortoiseshell, which were used to make such common items as combs and billiard balls. In fact, decades later in the 1940s, Henry Ford, who brought cars to the masses with the assembly line, developed a concept car made from soy-derived cellulose, but World War II put an end to its commercialization because of wartime rationing.

In 1907, the Belgian chemist Leo Baekeland made the world's first fully synthetic plastic, which he called Bakelite. Unlike cellulose, it was cheap to produce and could be molded into numerous objects, such as dishware, jewelry, clocks, telephones, and more. During World War II, synthetic plastics were mass-produced as substitutes for natural materials such as cork in life jackets and silk in parachutes. By the end of the war, the petrochemical industry was eager to stay in business, so they invented single-use plastic items for the home, such as plates, cutlery, and cups. These items came with the promise to consumers of convenience and freedom from household chores, and by the early 1960s, single-use plastic infiltrated everyday life. By the 1970s, by volume, plastic as a raw material was more widely used than aluminum or steel. In the mid-1980s, more than 100 million tons of plastic were produced, and by 2015 this amount had more than quadrupled to 448 million tons, with the bulk of it being used for packaging.

The Good

While single-use plastic is seemingly unavoidable nowadays, not all of its uses are bad. In the medical world, for example, plastic is an excellent material to use for incubators, tubes, and syringes to efficiently avoid cross-contamination. After a natural disaster, packaged items such as fresh water and nonperishable foods can save lives. When used in longer-life applications, such as in cars, laptops, and airplanes, plastic makes these items lighter and more durable and, therefore, more efficient.

The Bad

Half of all plastic produced becomes trash in less than a year. This lightweight, chemically toxic material never biodegrades but eventually breaks up into what are known as microplastics—fragments smaller than one-fifth of an inch (5 mm). These particles have reached every corner of the earth, from the highest mountains to the deepest seas, and are impossible to clean up.

The Ugly

Plastic waste is impacting our environment. Every piece of plastic ever made still exists in some shape or form in the air, on land, and in waterways and oceans. There are already an estimated 165 million tons of plastic in the ocean. Microplastics have infiltrated the food chain, from the phytoplankton that ingest the synthetic particles to the fish that feed on the plankton to eventually, the food on our plates. The chemical compounds found in plastic that are introduced into our bodies can cause hormonal imbalance, reproductive problems, nervous system damage, obesity, cancer, and heart disease. In addition, millions of animals are killed or injured every year by ingesting or becoming entangled in plastic debris. Petrochemical plants that produce the primary building blocks for plastic are often located in neighborhoods of color, where people suffer from a disproportionate number of cases of cancer and other health problems.

Greenwashing

Greenwashing is a deceptive way of marketing to promote a process or product that is said to be better for the environment but isn't always. In our efforts to be more eco-friendly, we have come to rely on these methods and materials.

- **RECYCLING**

  We've been led to believe that recycling is the solution to dealing with an accumulation of plastic, but only 9 percent of all the plastic ever made has been recycled. For the past few decades, many nations were sending their plastic refuse to China for recycling, but in 2017 the nation changed its policies. The following year the country enforced stricter and more rigorous standards because it became too expensive and difficult to recycle plastics that were often contaminated with food waste, mixed with other materials, or made of types of plastics that couldn't be recycled. With nowhere left to go, our plastic is being stockpiled, sent to landfills, incinerated, or winding up in our environment. The recycling process is complicated (see page 16), and manufacturers find it cheaper to make products out of virgin plastic pellets (called nurdles) than recycled plastic. In addition, items made from recycled plastic can only be recycled a handful of times; unlike glass and aluminum, the quality of plastic degrades with every iteration.

- **BIOPLASTICS**

  Bioplastics, materials made from plants such as corn or sugarcane, aren't all they're cracked up to be despite what we've been told; just because something is labeled biodegradable or compostable doesn't mean it will actually break down naturally. Sure they're made from biodegradable sources, but they require lots of land, water, pesticides, and fossil fuels to make and some take hundreds of years to biodegrade if not properly composted at an industrial facility—and even then they may never completely biodegrade. Easily confused for their synthetic counterparts, bioplastics are also often thrown into the recycling stream, rendering the whole batch unrecyclable.

- **PAPER**

  You're often faced with the choice: paper or plastic? The best answer is neither. Like bioplastics, paper products require a lot of resources to produce, and they can only be recycled between five and seven times. Plus, many paper products are coated with plastic to make them water-resistant, rendering them nonrecyclable.

- **SILICONE**

  Unlike plastic, silicone that is high quality and food grade is more stable when heated and is thought to be less likely to leach toxic chemicals into our food. It also has a longer useful life than ordinary plastic. Like plastic, silicone is made from fossil fuels, requires chemicals and carbon resources to produce, and never biodegrades. In addition, it can be difficult to find a recycling plant that will take silicone products, and more research is needed about the long-term effects of it on our health. Not all silicone is created equal, so we recommend looking for 100 percent food-grade silicone. Skip the brightly colored silicone and stick to clear colors, since colorants are often found to be a source of lead. If you do opt for hot pink, make sure the product label states "lead-free." Finally, avoid exposing silicone to high temperatures and opt for glass instead.

Solutions

As individuals, we can reduce plastic pollution by being conscious consumers. Zero waste can be cost effective and inclusive of all budgets. In order to reduce the world's plastic pollution, we collectively need to take action to end our reliance on this "disposable" material. If the world population of 7.8 billion people can make one plastic-free change each day, that's 7.8 billion pieces of plastic not used. Start with your own actions of refusing, reducing, and reusing plastic. This can inspire and educate others around you to do the same. The ripple effect in your community can also spark legislative action if enough people clamor for change.

- ### EDUCATION
  The first step is to acknowledge the problem and want to make a change. By picking up this book, you're already taking that step to become better informed and more

mindful of how our daily plastic habits are impacting not only our communities and health, but the entire planet. Knowing that there is no such thing as "disposable" plastic, the only way forward is to live without it.

- ## REFUSE, REDUCE, REUSE

Refuse to buy or use plastic, especially when you know that item will be heading to the trash can within a few minutes. Be mindful of situations in your daily life when you can "just say no" to plastic. Do you really need that bag, straw, or bottle? Think about selecting alternatives to these items. Reduce plastic usage by replacing these items with reusable products made from nontoxic materials, such as glass, cloth, or stainless steel. These steps help to avoid generating waste, forming a circular lifestyle of continuously reusing materials as opposed to a linear model of using something only once and then throwing it away.

- ## ACTIONS THROUGH LEGISLATION

Governments around the world are starting to take action to ban certain single-use plastics and require packaging to contain either minimum amounts of post-consumer recycled plastic or alternatives. You can call your local legislators and ask them to introduce bills to reduce plastic waste, such as banning plastic straws and bags.

TYPES OF PLASTIC

There are hundreds of types of plastics, but the following are most common. Ever wonder what those numbers, known as Resin Identification Codes (RIC), and chasing arrows on the bottom of your packaging really mean? Here's the key to decoding them. Check with your local recycling program, as every location has different procedures and rules.

RIC #	Name	Abbreviation	Common Use	Recyclability
1	Polyethylene terephthalate	PET or PETE	- Bottles for water, soft drinks, sports drinks, juice, mouthwash, and contact lens solution - Containers for condiments such as ketchup, peanut butter, and jelly - Trays that are microwavable - Film on microwavable trays - Certain clothes (polyester)	Accepted by most curbside programs
2	High-density polyethylene	HDPE	- Rigid: Bottles for milk, cleaning products, shampoo, laundry detergent, and cosmetics - Film: Bags for grocery/retail and for cereal box liners and other plastic films (any plastic 10 millimeters thick)	Bottles, containers, or other rigid packaging are accepted by most curbside programs. For bags and other films, take them to drop-off bins at major grocery and retail chains in the United States.

RIC #	Name	Abbreviation	Common Use	Recyclability
3	Polyvinyl chloride	PVC, Vinyl	- Food containers, including blister packs and clam shells - Shower curtains, bibs, purses, jackets, rain coats, and aprons	Isn't accepted by most curbside programs
4	Low-density polyethylene	LDPE	- Bags for bread, frozen foods, dry-cleaning and household garbage - Shrink wrap and cling film or coating on milk cartons and coffee cups - Bottles for condiments and lids for containers	Isn't accepted by most curbside programs, but is accepted at store drop-off programs found at major grocery and retail chains in the United States
5	Polypropylene	PP	- Containers for yogurt, cheese, and deli foods - Bottles for ketchup, syrup, prescriptions, and other condiments and medicines	Accepted by most curbside programs but has a low recycling rate
6	Polystyrene	PS	- Rigid or foamed: food-related items, such as cups, plates, bowls, coffee cup lids, containers (clamshells), and trays for prepackaged meat (Styrofoam)	Isn't accepted by most curbside programs
7	Other		- Every other plastic not listed here - Mixed plastics or combination of various bioplastics	Isn't accepted by most curbside programs

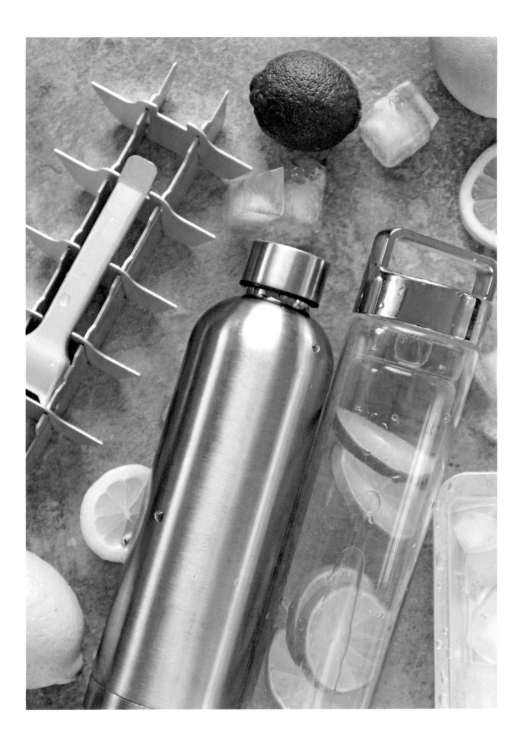

Start Now!

Don't despair—there's hope! Two simple changes you can make right now are ditching your plastic water bottles and plastic bags. It's easy!

WATER BOTTLES

Water is the source of life, but it's also the culprit for major plastic waste. And all of that waste is easy to avoid with one simple solution: the refillable water bottle.

It takes three liters of water to make a one-liter single-use plastic water bottle. For those of us fortunate enough to have access to clean, drinkable water, paying for water doesn't make any sense. Public drinking water facilities are required to test for contaminants each year and publicly disclose the results, while the bottled water industry is not required by law to disclose the results of its testing.

Whether at home or on the go, stay hydrated without all the plastic packaging by tapping into tap water. Use your own refillable glass or stainless-steel water bottle, cup, or jar. You can find places to refill your bottle using apps such as Tap and RefillMyBottle (see Resources, page 234), which share 34,000 refill stations across 7,100 cities in 30 countries. Never leave your house without a refillable bottle in your bag.

> **FACT** Americans throw away 35 billion plastic water bottles per year. Only one out of every five gets recycled.

BAGS

Just because a plastic bag is offered when you make a purchase doesn't mean you have to accept it. Reusable bags are lightweight and easy to stash. Always have one in your backpack or purse and maybe another two or three in your car. If you happen to forget your bag, skip it altogether and use your handbag, backpack, T-shirt, or hands.

Don't forget, it's not just grocery and shopping bags that are a problem. Produce bags (see page 98), food storage bags (see page 39), dry-cleaning garment bags (see page 56), dog poop bags (see page 52), and trash bags (see page 57) are also plastic offenders.

You can repurpose an old T-shirt into a reusable bag with only a pair of scissors. Lay the shirt flat on a table and cut off the sleeves at the seams. Draw a half circle with a dinner plate on the neckline (both front and back) then cut along the line. Along the bottom of the shirt, cut a fringe that is ½ inch wide by 5 inches long (1 cm × 12 cm). Tie each fringe with double knots.

> **FACT** An estimated 5 trillion plastic bags were used in 2019. That's equivalent to 160,000 bags a second. If you placed each bag side by side, they would wrap around the world seven times every hour and cover an area twice the size of France.

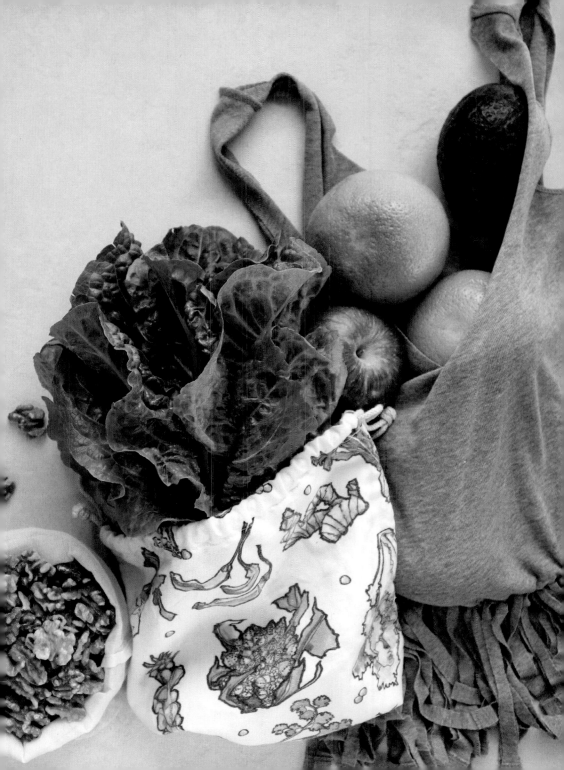

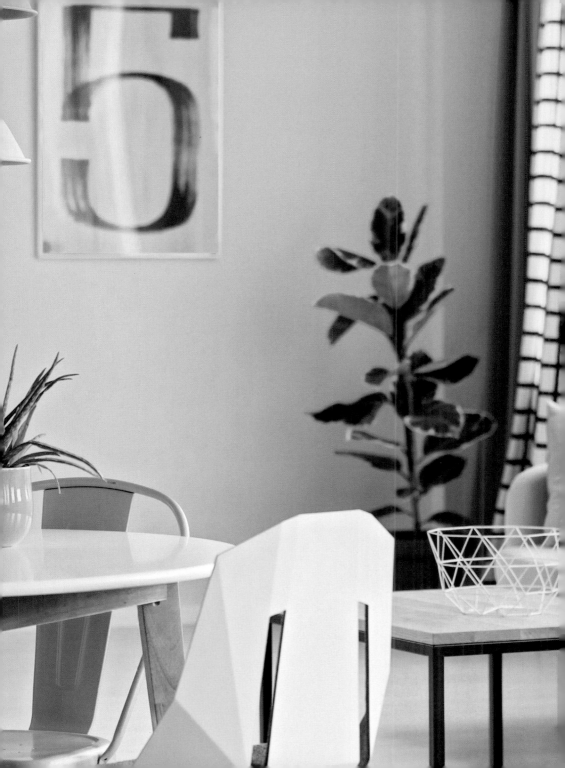

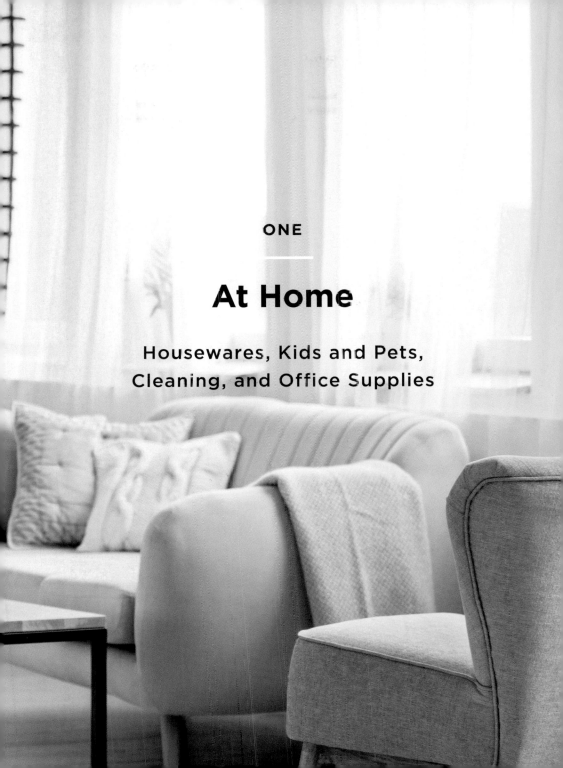

ONE

At Home

Housewares, Kids and Pets, Cleaning, and Office Supplies

Your home is a haven in which you spend the majority of your time. It's only common sense that you'd want its environment to promote your good health and well-being. Yet from your bedroom, where you spend a third of your life, to the kitchen, where you prepare meals, plastics can be found in almost everything. No matter where you live, whether a small apartment in the city or a large suburban or country home, keeping your environment clean and plastic-free is a matter of taking one step at a time.

This chapter examines plastic items that are used repeatedly in your home for many months, such as cutting boards or a blender. All plastics pose certain health risks, as they can leach or emit chemicals when subjected to repeated high temperatures or are cracked or scratched. Even plastics deemed safer than others have been found to leach chemicals when tested in laboratories under certain conditions. Instead of tossing and replacing every single plastic item you own, creating unnecessary waste, you can learn safer ways to use them to mitigate their negative impact on your health.

When it is time to buy new items for your home, consider things that are durable, like cast-iron pans, or that are naturally nontoxic, like a 100 percent organic hemp shower curtain that doesn't emit noxious fumes. Reverting back to the materials that people used before plastic became so ubiquitous is always a safe bet. While these items may be more expensive and require more care, they are designed to last and don't typically emit harmful chemicals.

MATTRESSES

One-third of your life is spent sleeping, so a good mattress is important. Rest at ease with mattresses made from biodegradable materials, including natural rubber latex, wool, coconut fiber, cotton, and even seaweed (see Resources, page 244)! These materials are inherently nonflammable, so they don't require any chemical flame retardants.

FACT Most mattresses are made of polyurethane foam (PU; RIC #7). Because this material is highly flammable, it's necessary for the manufacturers to add highly toxic flame retardants so the bed won't burst into flames. These chemicals are inhaled while you sleep and can cause respiratory and skin problems.

SHOWER CURTAINS

A shower curtain made from polyvinyl chloride (PVC) can be iden-
tified by the Resin Identification Code #3 and usually has a strong
plastic smell when new.

Buy an organic hemp or cotton shower curtain or get creative
and make your own from a repurposed cotton or linen bed sheet
or tablecloth. Make sure to wash a cloth curtain every few weeks
to avoid mildew. Or, for water-resistant protection, you can line the
cloth with beeswax (see page 41).

As for your old PVC (RIC #3) shower curtain, take it to your
local hazardous waste center. If you want to make a statement,
send it back to the manufacturer with a note asking them to switch
to safer materials.

FACT Shower curtains made from PVC contain toxic chemical additives
such as phthalates and lead to soften the material, which emit harmful
carcinogenic dioxins. In addition, these curtains aren't recyclable.

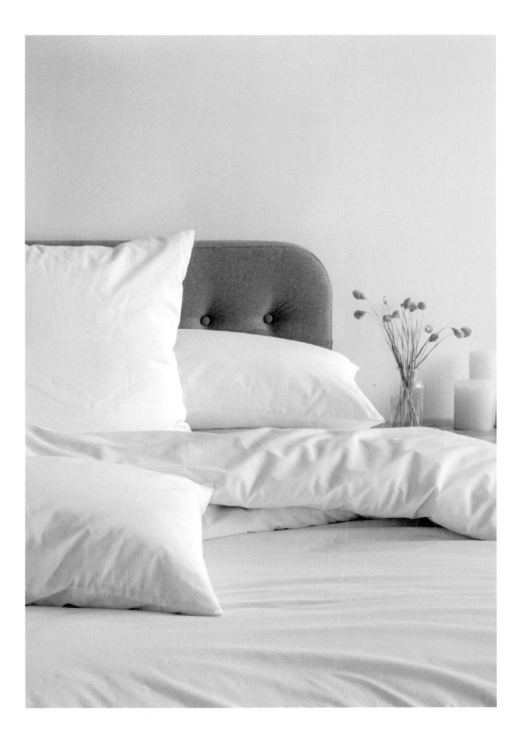

BED AND BATH LINENS

Read the labels to ensure that sheets, pillowcases, and bath towels aren't made from polyester blends. Look for 100 percent organic cotton, hemp, or bamboo.

Tencel lyocell fabrics are cellulose fibers made from sustainably sourced wood pulp that is produced in a closed-loop system where the materials used are recycled with minimal waste and low emissions. Like cotton and bamboo, Tencel is made from plant materials, so it is biodegradable. On top of that, Tencel requires less energy and water than cotton. It's also soft and breathable, so look for it in workout clothes. Brands like Patagonia and Reformation use it.

> **FACT** Cheap, synthetic (polyester, nylon, fleece, and sometimes flannel) bedding and towels aren't made to last, and microplastics are released when they're washed. They can also be uncomfortable to use because they aren't breathable like natural fibers.

CLOTHING

According to Greenpeace, wearing your clothes for at least two years will reduce greenhouse gas emissions by more than 24 percent. Buy pre-loved/pre-worn clothes to extend the useful life of clothes. Consignment options are plentiful and expected to surpass the luxury market by 2022.

When you buy new clothes, think quality over quantity and check the tag for 100 percent organic cotton, linen, hemp, bamboo, cashmere, silk, and wool. These natural materials are more durable.

Remember that when you wash synthetic clothes, microfibers (smaller than the diameter of a hair) are flushed into the ocean, so consider washing them in a Guppyfriend washing bag (see Resources, page 235); it's currently the only way to try to filter microplastics in top-load washing machines.

Wash your clothes less frequently, too. And when you do, select cold water, run a full load, and use liquid DIY soap or soap nuts (see page 235).

FACT Clothing can be repaired, repurposed into other items (make rags or bags, or alter long sleeves to tanks tops and jeans into shorts), or recycled (wool and cotton), and yet more than 11 million tons of clothing, shoes, and textiles are sent to landfills each year.

KITCHEN APPLIANCES

Plastic is everywhere in your kitchen—in the refrigerator's produce drawers, in your blender and food processor bowls, and in a plethora of other gadgets. It would be costly to replace all these items, so you should try to minimize the time that your food comes in contact with plastic.

For instance, lining refrigerator produce drawers with a cotton bath towel will not only provide a barrier between the vegetables and the plastic, it will also keep veggies fresher longer.

Hand-wash plastics, even if they are said to be dishwasher safe, because extreme heat can cause phthalates and Bisphenol A (BPA) to leach out. By the same token, ensure that whatever food you place in a blender or food processor has sufficiently cooled before using.

KITCHEN COOKWARE

Avoid Teflon nonstick pans, and instead choose a well-seasoned cast-iron pan with a natural oil coating. It'll perform just as well as a nonstick pan. Enameled cast-iron cookware from Le Creuset or Lodge are heavy-duty and well worth the investment because of their durability. Stainless steel is another tried-and-true material for cooking. For baking, opt for classic heatproof glass or ceramic pans.

FACT The birth of Teflon happened in 1938 when a slippery white solid plastic compound, polytetrafluoroethylene (PTFE; RIC #7), was discovered. Combined with polyfluoroalkyl and perfluoroalkyl compounds (PFAs; RIC #7), the first Teflon products were sold in 1946 touting an innovative slippery surface that keeps food from sticking when cooking and baking. If any of your Teflon cookware has been scratched, it's best not to use it, as the coating will continue to chip off, leaching into your food.

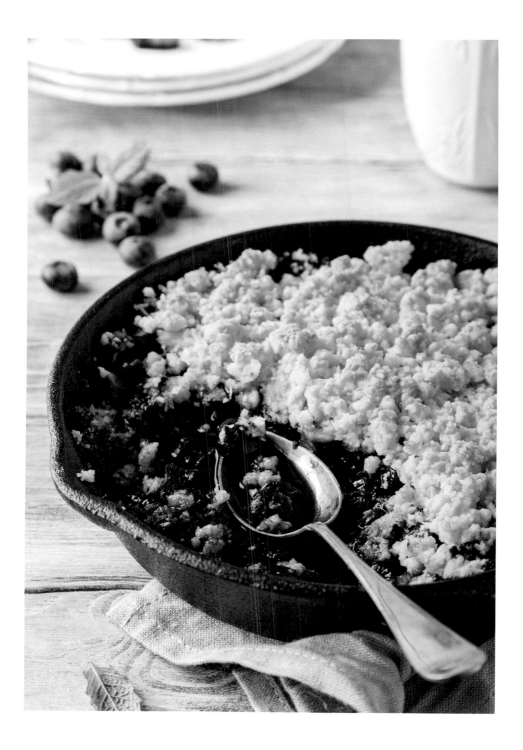

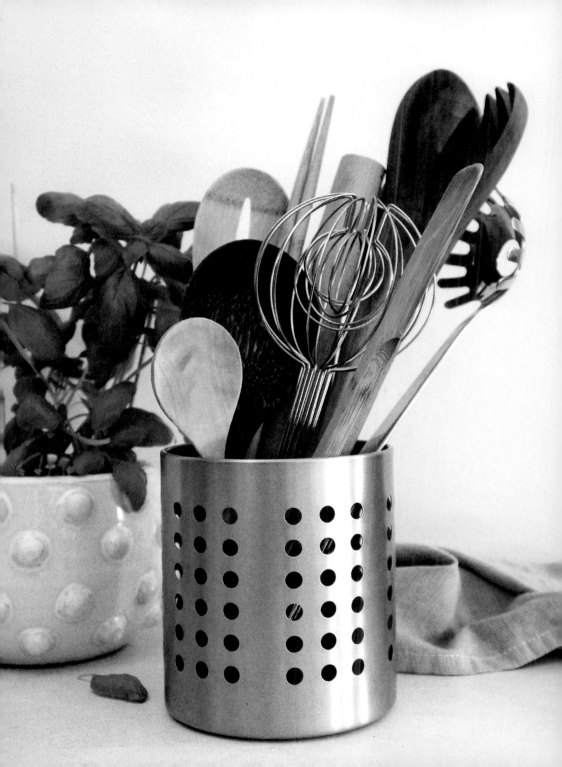

KITCHEN UTENSILS

Wooden or bamboo cooking tools are handy for hot foods and great because they don't scratch cookware surfaces. Always hand wash and air-dry these items to prevent them from cracking. Rub with coconut oil once a week to maintain these utensils.

> **FACT** Nylon cooking tools can melt or flake off with continued use, which can contaminate your food. Plastic utensils, particularly black ones, have been found to contain traces of brominated flame retardants, chlorine, cadmium, chromium, mercury, and lead.

CUTTING BOARDS

Use a hard wood or bamboo cutting board that doesn't have any synthetic coatings or glues. Wood is a safe choice because it has natural antibacterial properties, and continuous usage won't damage the board. Maintain your cutting board by giving it a good salt scrub once a month: evenly sprinkle coarse salt on the surface then scrub it with half a lemon, squeezing some of the juice out as you scrub. Let this rest for 5 minutes before rinsing the board with hot water. When dry, treat it with a coat of almond or walnut oil.

FACT When slicing produce, bread, or meat on a plastic cutting board, you're likely cutting deep grooves into the surface. These scratches are not only breeding grounds for bacteria, they also can release pieces of plastic, or microplastics, directly into your food.

WATER FILTERS

Activated charcoal is the purifying ingredient commonly found in water filters. Pure, naked charcoal sticks (see Resources, page 234) make an excellent water purifier, without any plastic. It's a piece of wood, typically oak, that has been heated in an extremely hot kiln, which carbonizes the stick into 97 percent carbon. Carbon naturally bonds with toxins, absorbing the metals found in tap water such as lead, mercury, copper, and aluminum.

To use, rinse and boil a stick or sticks for five minutes, and let the charcoal dry out in the sunshine for an hour. Then simply place the stick(s) in a glass jug and fill it with tap water. Once a month, keep the charcoal sticks active by repeating the process. After four months of use, turn these sticks into an air freshener in your refrigerator, closet, bathroom, or car. You can also crush the charcoal and use it as biochar in your plants or garden to improve the soil and encourage plant growth.

FACT Globally, the consumption of bottled water continues to grow each year, reaching almost 100 billion gallons (373.5 billion L) in 2017.

NAPKINS AND TOWELS

Wipe up a mess with reusable, more durable cotton dish cloths, towels, napkins, and rags.

You can even make your own "unpaper" towel roll. Cut up an old sheet into your desired size and hem the edges with a zigzag stitch. Sew two pieces together for a two-ply towel. Roll them up and store in a handy wide-mouthed jar for easy access.

FACT Americans spend more on paper towels than the combined sum of the rest of the world.

Aside from being packaged in flimsy, difficult to recycle plastic, paper towels and napkins have been shown to contain traces of BPA (RIC #7) and Bisphenol S (BPS; RIC #7), because thermal paper (see page 164) gets recycled with paper products.

FOOD STORAGE

Stop buying and collecting single-use food bags, cling film, and takeout containers. Reusable glass containers and jars are great for meal prep and for storing leftovers. When freezing liquids, make sure to fill the jar only three-quarters of the way full to allow for expansion and avoid breakage. Thaw overnight in the refrigerator before reheating.

Portion leftovers out for a convenient grab-and-go lunch. Stainless-steel containers are great for durability, especially with little ones, or to take on the go.

Plastic food bags can be replaced with certified compostable If You Care unbleached bags, Stasher Bags silicone storage bags, LunchSkins reusable zippered bags, or fun compostable paper sandwich bags (see Resources, page 237).

FACT In 1938, businessman and inventor Earl Tupper developed a durable plastic material made from oil refinement waste, Poly-T, which he used to create products for food storage. By the mid-1950s, thanks to Tupperware parties, they became household staples to store food. Although meant for reuse, similar "disposable" lightweight plastic food packaging is now common in the food industry for takeout and food delivery. Heat, acid, and oil from foods can leach into the plastic (and vice versa), as evidenced when stains and odors linger in a plastic food container. Never microwave food in plastic.

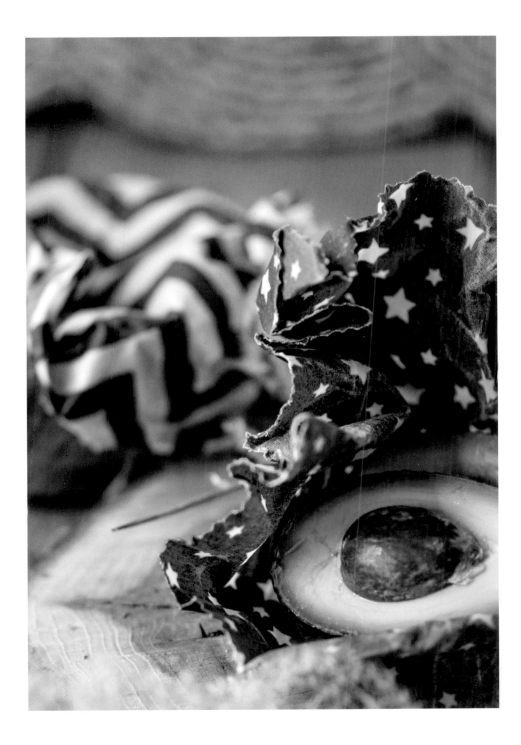

WAX FOOD WRAPS

Skip the plastic wrap and simply keep your leftovers covered with a plate, bowl, or cookware lid. For baking, when letting dough rest, wrap it with parchment paper or cover the bowl with a damp tea towel. Beeswax wraps, made of cotton coated with beeswax and natural oils, can be used as a substitute for plastic wrap. They can hold sandwiches and cover foods. You can also sew them to make handy snack bags.

WHAT YOU'LL NEED

1 yard (91 cm) 100 percent cotton fabric (organic, if possible)

Iron and ironing board

Parchment paper, larger than the fabric swatches

Cardboard, larger than the fabric swatches

2 to 3 teaspoons beeswax or non-GMO soy wax

Wash and dry the fabric to preshrink it. Cut the fabric into the desired shapes and sizes. For example, for smaller fruits cut in half, such as lemons and avocados, 7 × 7 inches (18 × 18 cm); to wrap a sandwich, 13 × 13 inches (33 × 33 cm), and to cover a large bowl, 16 × 16 inches (40 × 40 cm). Use sewing scissors for a clean cut or fabric scissors with a sawtooth edge.

(continued)

Iron your fabric swatches to remove wrinkles, then turn the iron down to its lowest, no-steam setting. Put a large piece of cardboard onto your ironing board and place a piece of parchment paper on top of this. Put the first piece of fabric onto the parchment paper. Lightly and evenly sprinkle granules of the wax onto the fabric, making sure to cover the edges and corners. It doesn't need to be a thick layer because once heated, the wax will melt and spread. Place another piece of parchment paper on top of the fabric and iron the parchment until the wax has melted into the fabric. Take care to not directly iron any stray wax granules. When the wax has melted, peel the parchment paper off the fabric and check for any uncoated spots. If there are any, sprinkle more wax on the uncoated spots and repeat the melting process. Hang the fabric up to dry.

To clean the wraps, simply wash with cool water and dish soap and let them air-dry. Refresh your wraps by melting more wax onto them.

FACT Aside from the fact that cling film never degrades, studies have found that there are 175 compounds in it, including BPA (RIC #7). The amount of plastic wrap Americans use every year could cover Texas!

BABY BOTTLES

If breastfeeding isn't possible, use glass bottles. Glass is easy to sanitize in the dishwasher and for heating milk on the stovetop.

Choose baby bottle nipples made from medical-grade silicone instead of synthetic latex to avoid a volatile compound called N-nitrosamines, which can be formed during the manufacturing process. Be sure to hand wash and replace before they start wearing down.

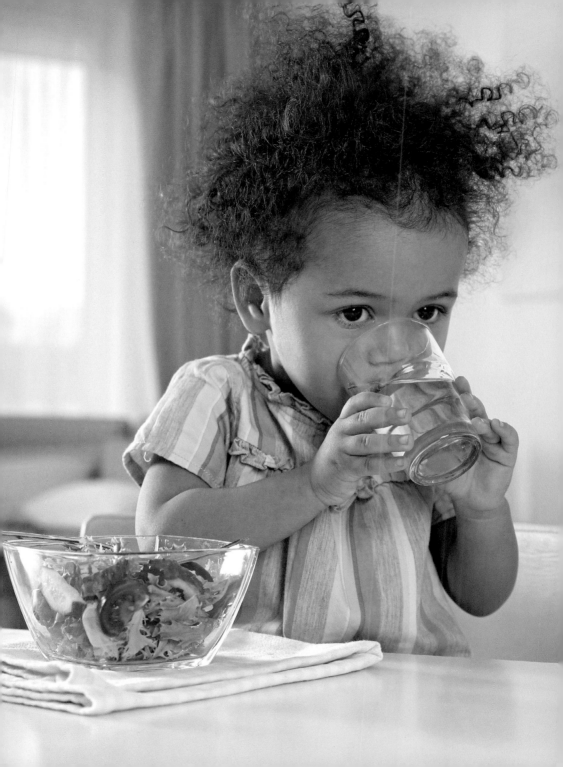

KIDS' TABLEWARE AND CUPS

Skip the sippy. Experts say that sippy cups can damage teeth and delay oral motor skills such as learning how to swallow, which is integral to progressing to solid foods. Wean babies off the bottle with an open glass or stainless-steel cup with a soft silicone round lip or straw instead.

Once your toddler starts eating solid foods, use high-quality coconut bowls and stainless-steel plates for durability. As your child gets older and you migrate to ceramic dishes and glassware, it's the perfect opportunity to explain why you are not using plastic, even though it is colorful (and durable and inexpensive). This also helps them learn how to properly care for things that break easily, an important lifelong lesson.

FACT While a sippy cup is convenient for parents and can appease babies and toddlers, the hard plastic, which gets chewed and scuffed over time, can be ingested and absorbed through the baby's skin. BPA-free does not mean that it is safe, as the BPS or other replacement chemicals can also cause hormonal, behavioral, and developmental imbalances.

BABY PRODUCTS

A child's skin absorbs toxins more easily than an adult's, and children are much more apt to get toxic substances in their bodies both through touch and by putting things in their mouths. From rubberwood bath toys to bamboo bibs to 100 percent organic wool puddle pads (mattress protectors), natural, nontoxic, plastic-free alternatives can be found for your baby (see Resources, page 234).

> **FACT** According to the Environmental Working Group (EWG), children use an average of five personal care products every day and are exposed to an average of sixty-one unique ingredients in these products each day, twenty-seven of which are unsafe. Many baby bibs are made from vinyl (PVC), which should be avoided.

BABY WIPES

Clean baby's little fingers, toes, and tushy with reusable cloth wipes. Whether at home or on the go, have a stack of dry cloths on hand and wet them with water, if necessary. Make sure to carry a separate bag to hold all your soiled cloth wipes (and diapers) and toss them in the wash when the bag is full.

FACT Aside from the plastic packaging they come in, wet wipes are neither reusable nor recyclable. Most are made with polyester or polypropylene, and as with any products with fragrance, they contain chemicals called phthalates, also known as "plasticizers." Overuse of chemical wipes can actually weaken immune systems and increase chances of allergies and "superbugs" or antibiotic-resistant bacteria.

DIAPERS

Purchase a selection of reusable cloth diapers to see which option works for you. There are a variety of inserts and covers available in cotton, hemp, and bamboo. Wool, which is naturally waterproof, is often used for reusable diaper covers.

If you're feeling overwhelmed with laundry and a newborn, using a diaper service can help, but it's more economical to wash the diapers at home. Soak and wash diapers first in a warm short cycle to rinse away the surface soil. Then run a full hot-water wash. Drying them in the sunshine is also a great option to keep diapers clean, as the sun kills dust mites and odors.

FACT "Disposable" diapers, launched in 1949, are made of a mix of plastic compounds like nylon, polyester, polyethylene, polypropylene, polyurethane foam, and/or Lycra. Globally, 450 billion single-use disposable diapers are used each year, contributing to 77 million tons of solid waste in landfills in the United States alone—*ew*!

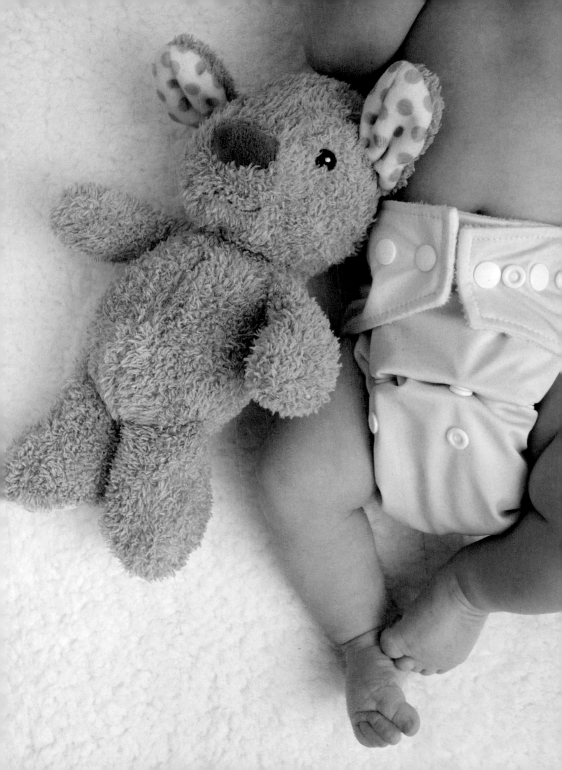

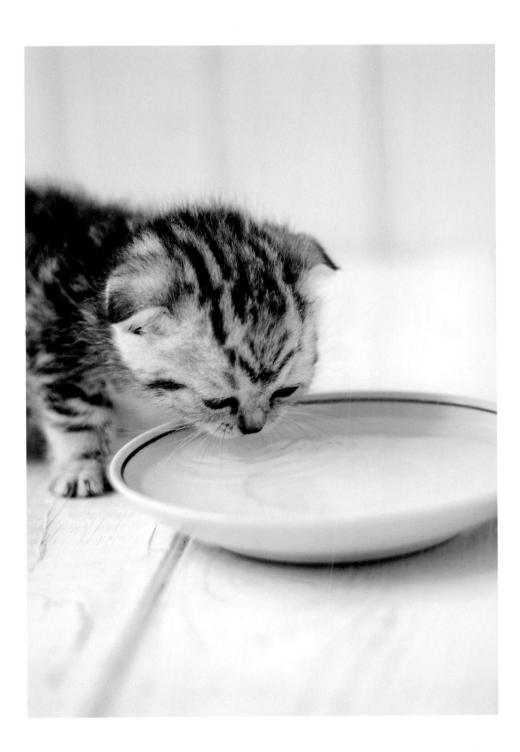

PET FOOD

Buy dry pet food that comes in compostable paper/cardboard packaging. Some pet stores sell it in bulk, which you can carry home in your own container. You can also make your own pet food and treats. When serving the food, use ceramic or stainless-steel bowls.

FACT As with humans, it is best to limit your pet's exposure to plastic. PVC (RIC #3) or BPA/BPS (RIC #7) coating lines the cans and packaging of most common pet food.

DOG WASTE

When your dog is ready to go, slip some newspaper or scrap paper underneath for the poop to land on. For any accidents or incidents close to or at home, dog poop can be flushed or composted in a pet waste "toilet." In some cities, there are also dedicated pet waste collection facilities.

CAT WASTE

DIY kitty litter can be as simple as using sawdust, sand, or mulch. Integrity is a brand of natural litter made from a mix of wheat with aspen (see Resources, page 235). Add some baking soda to control odors.

And never flush your cat's waste. Cat poop can contain a protozoan parasite called *Toxoplasmosis gondii*, which comes from contact with wild animals or eating raw meat and is harmful to humans and marine life. Wastewater facilities can't remove this parasite, so there is a chance it could be released into the environment.

PET ACCESSORIES

Animals in the wild don't need toys, but to keep indoor domesti-
cated animals stimulated mentally and physically they can use a few
playthings. Our pets are sensitive to man-made chemicals, too, so
opt for natural and compostable materials, or make your own toys
out of old jeans, T-shirts, or towels. Whether buying or making your
own toys, look for items that are made to last.

FACT A typical pet store is filled with plastic toys, balls, travel carriers,
and habitats for our furry and feathered friends. There aren't any
government regulations for these items, and studies have found many to
contain PVC (RIC #3), phthalates, BPA (RIC #7), and toxic heavy metals.

LAUNDRY

Clean your clothes with the power of nuts. Horse chestnuts (aka buckeyes or conkers), which are commonly found in forests and backyards in the Western hemisphere, make a great laundry cleaner. Prepare a detergent for one load of laundry by placing five chestnuts into an old towel and cracking them open with a hammer into small pieces, or simply slice them into quarters. Place the pieces into a dedicated detergent glass jar, fill it with boiling hot water, and leave overnight. The next day, remove the chestnuts from the liquid. (Save the fully dried chestnut solids to prepare another two batches of detergent.) Store the liquid in an airtight jar in the refrigerator for up to a week. Use ½ cup (120 ml) of this milky liquid per load of laundry.

Soap nuts, also known as soapberries, are related to the lychee fruit and contain saponin, a natural cleaning agent. They come from *Sapindus mukorossi* trees, which typically grow in northern India and Nepal, but you can order soap nuts online (see Resources, page 235). Simply place five soap nuts into a small cloth bag (or a thin sock) that can be tied up tightly and throw the bag into the washer with your dirty laundry. You can use each bundle five times and compost them afterward.

If you must buy commercially made detergent, look for one that comes in a cardboard box. Try to find a brand that doesn't include a plastic liner or scoop in every box.

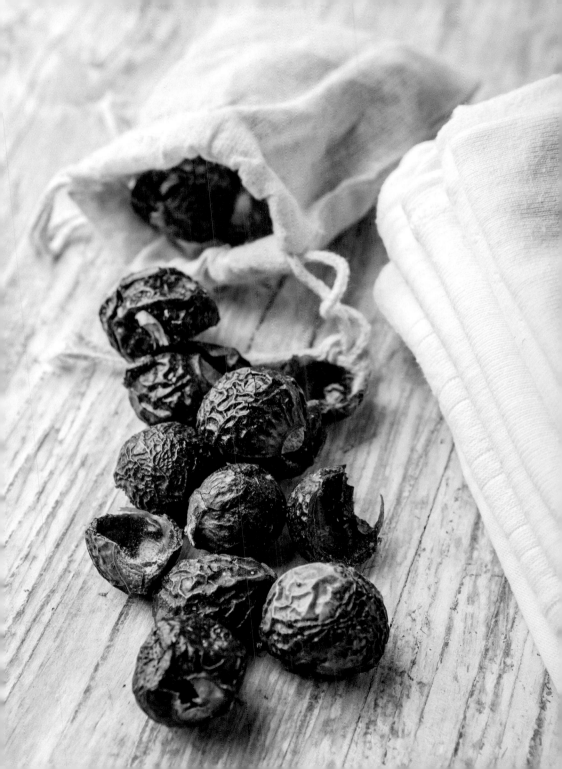

DRY CLEANING

Gently hand wash, brush, or steam garments to keep them clean. For garments that need a little deodorizing, lightly spritz the fabric with vodka to kill off the odor-causing bacteria; just don't use it on delicate fabrics like silk.

Direct sunshine is also nature's disinfectant, keeping clothing free from dust mites and odors. Expose each side of the garment for thirty minutes.

If you must dry clean an article of clothing, make sure to also drop off a reusable garment bag for the dry cleaner to package your clean garment.

FACT Single-use plastic film dry-cleaning bags could be yellowing your clothes because they trap the cleaning chemicals. Worse yet, these bags add 300 million pounds of waste to US landfils each year.

TRASH BAGS

Forty percent of household waste is composed of food scraps. Setting up an at-home compost system (see page 65) or taking your food scraps to a community composting place and responsibly recycling them means there will be less trash winding up in a landfill and you'll use fewer plastic trash bags. When you take these steps, your trash will be mostly dry (no food moisture or mess), which means you won't need to line your trash cans with plastic at all.

Bioplastic trash bags should be better for the environment by virtue of their nonpetroleum renewable-based feedstock, but they require an industrial composting facility in order to properly biodegrade. There's also no telling if harmful additives or chemicals were added during the manufacturing process, and not all bags labeled biodegradable or compostable will actually break down in a compost facility.

When you get really efficient at reducing waste, you might be able to collect a year's worth of trash in something as small as a mason jar!

> **FACT** The first plastic garbage bag was produced in 1950. Globally, these bags collect 7.4 million tons of waste each day from households, schools, offices, businesses, farms, and other sources.

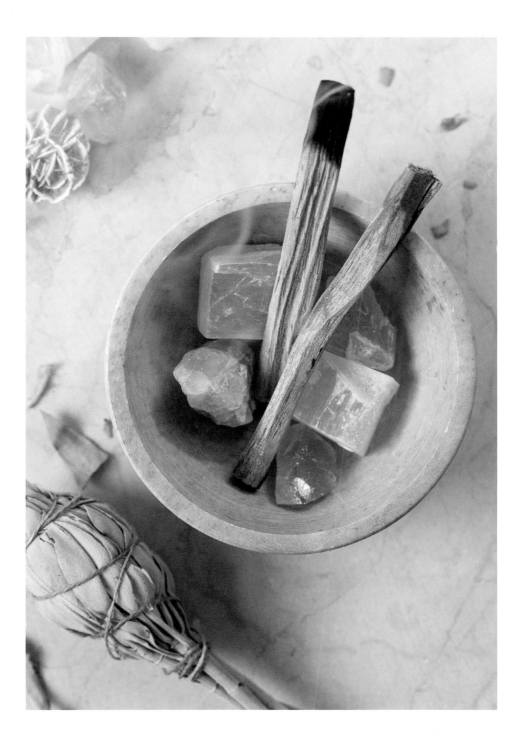

AIR FRESHENERS

Purify the air in your home with plants. Houseplants such as bamboo palm, spider plants, English ivy, chrysanthemums, aloe vera, and mother-in-law's tongue can keep the air clean and free from the toxic compounds that accumulate indoors. Aroma sprays and mists, essential oil diffusers, and herbal incense smudge sticks such as sage and palo santo wood can also clear the air.

You can also make your own natural room spray. In a glass spray bottle, combine ½ cup (120 ml) water with 1 tablespoon of vodka, 2 teaspoons of baking soda, and 10 drops of your favorite essential oil, such as lavender or citrus.

Give your living space a breath of fresh air by throwing open the windows whenever the weather allows.

FACT Studies have found that twelve out of fourteen air fresheners in the United States contain phthalates, chemicals used to dissolve and carry fragrances. These can cause a number of health concerns, including hormonal and reproductive issues, birth defects, and developmental disorders.

SPONGES

To scrub-a-dub-dub, look for pure cellulose sponges or natural ones from the sea or grown in nature. Did you know that a loofah actually comes from the fruit of a plant? The luffa is a tropical gourd that is part of the cucumber family. The young fruits can be eaten, but when allowed to mature and dry out, the skin is peeled off to reveal a perfect nonabrasive sponge that really gets the job done!

To keep your loofah longer, make sure it dries out thoroughly after each use, and clean it every two weeks by soaking it in 2 cups (475 ml) warm water mixed with 1 tablespoon baking soda for fifteen minutes. Squeeze out the water and let the loofah air-dry in a well-ventilated spot.

Wooden brushes and scrubbers or cotton washcloths are also great alternatives to synthetic sponges.

FACT The most common synthetic sponges are made from cellulose with a blend of polyester, polyurethane, or foamed plastic polymers. With regular use, these break down into pieces that go down the drain.

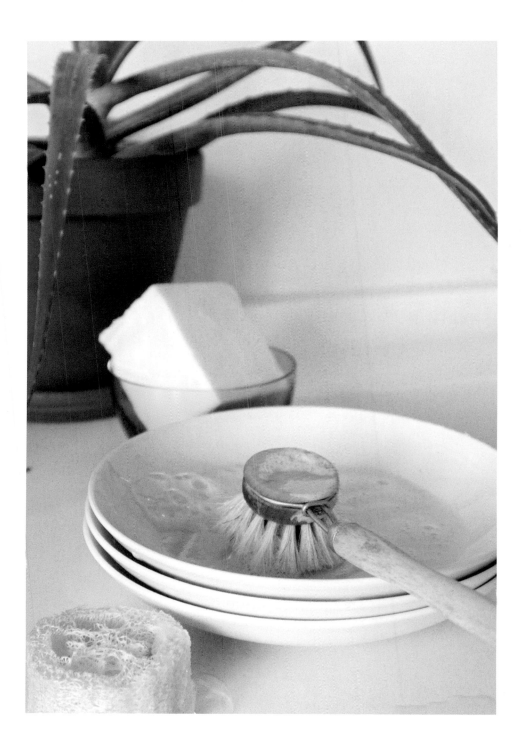

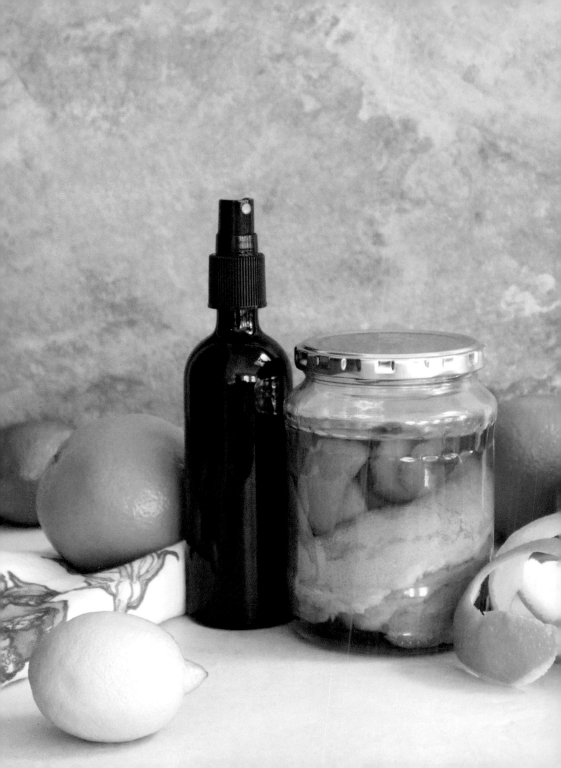

CLEANING PRODUCTS

Prepare your own cleaning products with only a few basic ingredients. For a good all-purpose cleanser, mix one part distilled white vinegar to three parts water. Baking soda (bicarbonate of soda) is a great natural deodorizer and scouring powder.

You can also make a refreshing, grease-cutting citrus cleanser by using discarded orange and lemon peels. Collect the peels in a 16-ounce (490 ml) jar stored in in the freezer. When the jar is full, fill it with distilled white vinegar, close the lid, and store in a dark spot (like under your kitchen sink) for two weeks. Take the peels out (and compost them!), then mix one part of this citrus-vinegar solution with one part water in a spray bottle to clean your kitchen or bathroom surfaces.

FACT Most glass, tile, and stainless-steel cleansers contain polyurethane, and toilet cleansers can contain polyester/polyamide and acrylic. These are plastics that act as abrasive scrubbing agents and are harmful to the environment when they enter the water system.

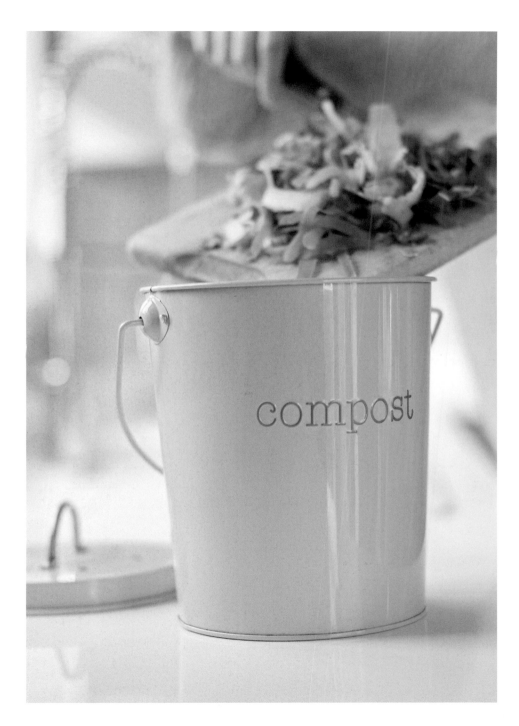

COMPOSTING

A home composter is a great way to both utilize food scraps and make nutrients for your soil. It also eliminates the need for a plastic trash bag.

Collect food scraps (vegetables, fruits, coffee grounds, eggshells, and bread) and unbleached paper products so they can be recycled back into the earth. Use a stainless-steel or ceramic container with a tight seal and keep it on your kitchen counter, under the sink, or in the freezer. You can also use a worm composter, a galvanized steel compost tumbler, or the FoodCycler, a handy kitchen appliance (see Resources, page 236). Don't add meat, dairy, or fish when composting at home to avoid attracting unwanted pests. Never compost grease and oils.

If you aren't able to compost at home, try finding a composting center, community garden, co-op, or a farmers' market to drop off your food scraps. Just be sure to follow their list of acceptable composting items.

> **FACT** By reducing the amount of food scraps sent to a landfill, you are helping to reduce methane gas emissions. Food waste in landfills is packed in with nonorganic waste and lacks the proper space, temperature, and moisture to degrade. The waste will never break down. Instead it produces methane gas, a harmful greenhouse gas.

HOME ENTERTAINMENT

Instead of watching DVDs or purchasing CDs, stream your favorite movies and music via on-demand or subscription services. Video games can also be purchased electronically or downloaded as an app on a device.

Sell your CDs, DVDs, laser discs, MP3s, VHS tapes, and any other systems on websites like Second Spin or eBay, or send them to the CD Recycling Center of America or GreenDisk (see Resources, page 235). Of course, consider hanging on to that limited-edition DVD if you think it might be a collector's item one day.

FACT DVDs are made from a brittle plastic called polycarbonate with a middle layer of aluminum that's covered by another layer of plastic. Because of these mixed layers, DVDs are classified as "other" plastic (RIC #7), and are not accepted by most curbside recyclers.

ELECTRONICS

To reduce your e-waste impact, opt to buy used or refurbished electronics. Always try to fix what you have before considering an upgrade. And donate, sell, or return your electronics to the manufacturer when you buy new ones. Some companies have an exchange policy in which they offer a rebate when you turn in your old gadget when purchasing a newer version.

Know where and how to responsibly recycle your e-waste with companies like the Electronics TakeBack Coalition or TerraCycle (see Resources, page 235).

FACT E-waste is a growing problem and harmful to the environment. Globally, only 15 percent of electronics gets recycled, and 20 percent of this waste is made up of polychlorinated biphenyls (PCBs).

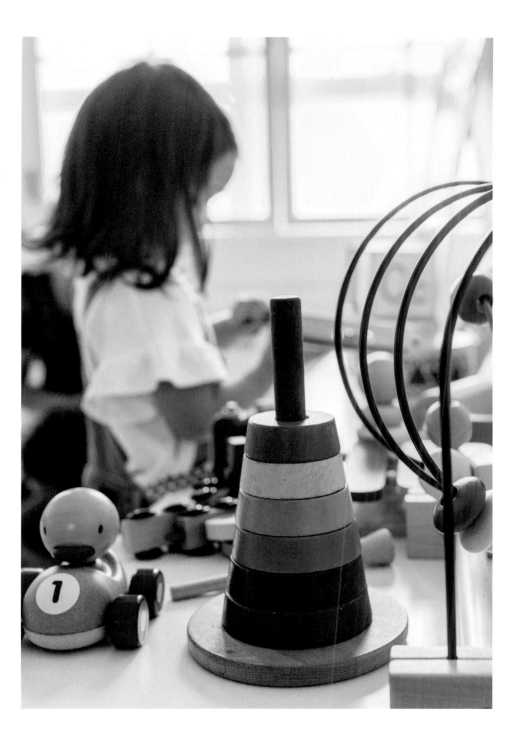

TOYS AND GAMES

Keep it simple with toys that allow creativity and imagination. Wooden blocks, cloth books made from organic cotton fabric swatches, musical instruments (even pots and pans!), paper, crayons, and board games can provide hours of entertainment. Look for durable toys made from wood, cotton, or natural rubber; they'll last longer.

Cute plushies made of and filled with certified organic, non-toxic materials can be found at Bears for Humanity, Under the Nile, and Elly Lu Organics (see Resources, page 235). Remember the sock monkey? Try making a homemade sewn doll or knitting animals and stuffing them with cut-up old clothing scraps or cotton or wool batting.

FACT Plastic toys, which tend to be inexpensive and vibrantly colored, account for 90 percent of the toy market. While they pose the same risks as any other plastic items in terms of exposure to chemicals, these playthings often have short life spans and are nearly impossible to recycle.

Plush toys are often made with synthetic fabrics like polyester and also stuffed with polystyrene foam beads or polyester batting. While soft and cuddly, these stuffed animals are also laced with chemical flame retardants.

ARTS AND CRAFTS

Make your own watercolor paint with food.

WHAT YOU'LL NEED

For Yellow: 2 small golden beets (120 g)

For Orange: 2 carrots (100 g)

For Red: 1 small beet (120 g)

For Green: 1 cup (120 g) spinach

Juice each vegetable separately in a juicer; be sure to rinse the machine in between each color creation.

Place each juice in its own small jar and add 1 teaspoon of white vinegar to each jar. Dip your paintbrush in and paint. If you want softer colors, you can dilute the mixtures with more water. Store in the refrigerator for 1 to 2 weeks.

Makes ⅓ cup (80 ml) of each color.

FACT Kids' paints, even the nontoxic ones, are made from chemicals, including polymers and phthalates that are easily absorbed through a child's sensitive skin.

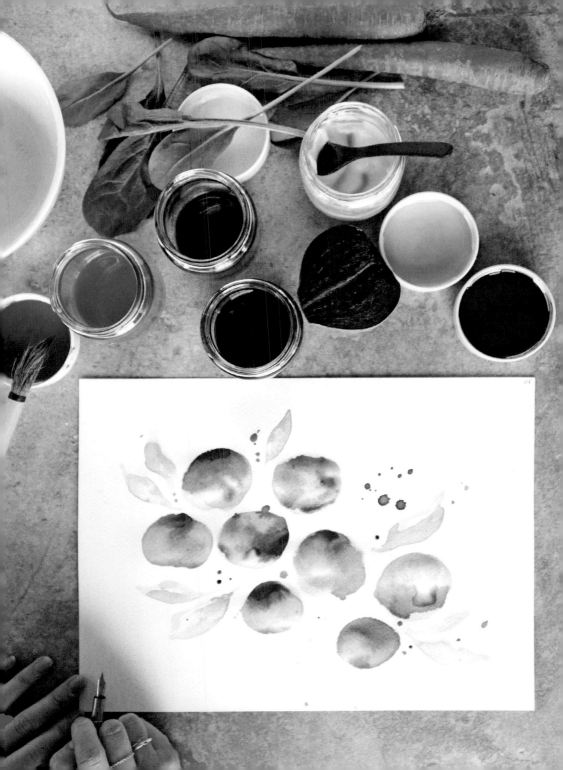

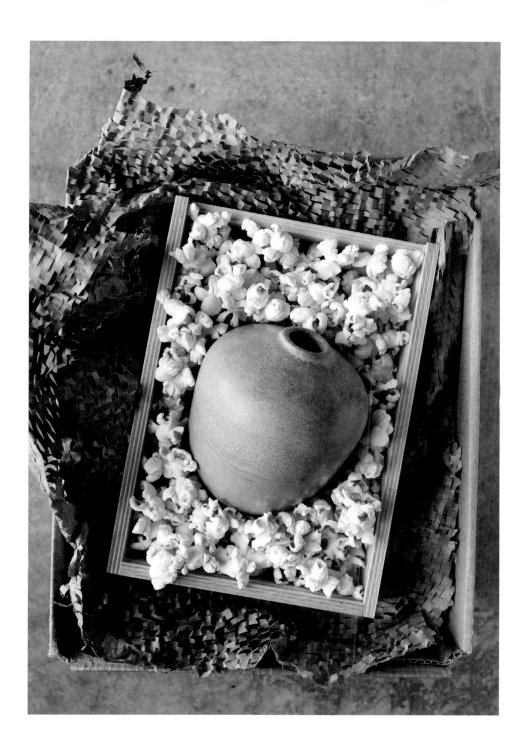

PACKING MATERIALS

Instead of using plastic packaging materials, including those annoying polystyrene peanuts, fill your shipping and gift boxes with crumpled newspapers, shredded paper, or used gift wrap. Plain popped popcorn, from the bulk bin section of your grocery store, also makes a great filler.

Use sustainable packing material, such as Geami (see Resources, page 236), a patented wrap made of craft and tissue paper, as an alternative to conventional bubble wrap. To avoid receiving bubble wrap/air cushions, buy from retailers that are committed to using minimal packaging (see Resources, page 233).

Companies like Lush Cosmetics use corn-based packing peanuts, a biodegradable and nontoxic alternative that dissolves when placed in water. Dell and Ikea are starting to use mushroom foam designed by Ecovative (see Resources, page 236), which is 100 percent compostable at home.

FACT Polystyrene peanuts pose a significant problem in landfills because they are so lightweight and easily escape by wind or are carried away by animals. The peanuts constitute 15 percent of the litter found in waterways, storm drains, and marine environments.

MAILING ENVELOPES

Use 100 percent recycled padded pulp paper envelopes, which can be recycled again or composted (see Resources, page 236). You can also reuse old mailers by covering up the previous address with paper and biodegradable cellulose tape, or reuse them to store fragile items.

If you receive a plastic bubble mailer with a paper address label, remove the label before recycling.

FACT Bubble wrap, originally invented in 1957, was intended to be used as wallpaper but instead became a widely used packaging material to protect items in transit. As online sales have increased, air cushions are used more frequently than any other material because they are the most cost-effective. Curbside recycling programs don't accept bubble wrap made from low-density polyethylene (LDPE; RIC #4) and air cushions made from high-density polyethylene (HDPE; RIC #2) because they get caught in the machinery at the material recovery facility. However, it is possible to recycle them along with plastic bags at many grocery stores and pharmacies in the United States.

PRINTER CARTRIDGES

Toner and ink cartridges are refillable, some even up to six times. Retailers such as Costco will refill them for a fraction of the cost of buying a new one. If you refill them at home, be prepared to get messy. You can also look for cartridges made from post-consumer recycled plastic.

When a cartridge has reached the end of its useful life, recycle it at Staples, OfficeMax, or Office Depot locations in the United States.

FACT It takes over 1 gallon (3.78 L) of oil to manufacture the printer cartridge, so reusing your cartridge even four times equals a savings of 3 gallons (11.3 L) of oil. That's enough gas to drive 70 miles (112 km), the distance between Miami and Palm Beach.

PENS

Buy a new or used fountain pen that can be refilled with ink from a glass jar. A fountain pen might seem like a big investment up front, but it's more cost-effective in the long run and much gentler on the environment. Make sure to find a refill converter so you can reuse your cartridge. Writing with a fountain pen can also be easier on the hand because less pressure is needed for the ink to come out, once you get the hang of it.

FACT In the early 1950s, the French company Bic mass-produced the first disposable ballpoint pen made from clear polystyrene. By 2005, Bic had sold more than 100 billion ballpoint pens globally, which is equivalent to the combined average weight of over four thousand adult male blue whales.

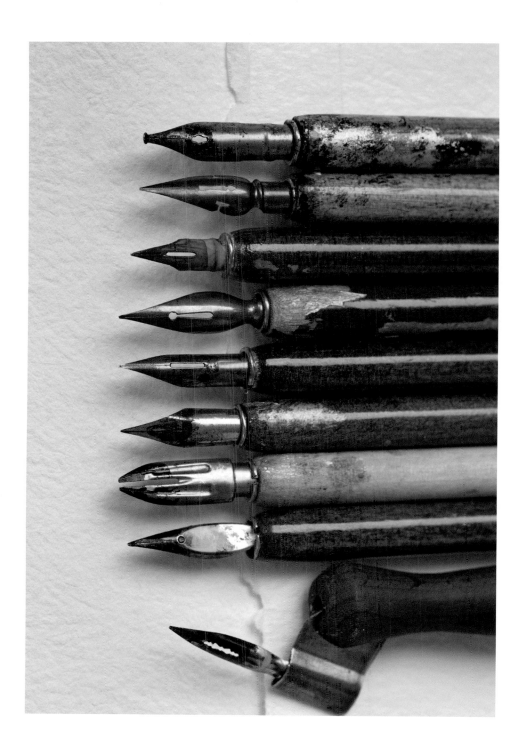

TAPE

Choose from three 100 percent biodegradable tapes.

- Cellulose is a natural byproduct of wood, mixed with a natural rubber adhesive (as opposed to synthetic resin adhesives). This tape is strong and transparent, so it seals boxes and weatherproofs labels.
- Gummed paper tape is a water-activated tape with a layer of kraft paper and rubber adhesive.
- Masking tape made from crepe paper and a rubber adhesive is good for sealing envelopes. (See Sources, page 245.)

FACT Scotch Tape, initially manufactured by 3M in 1925, was the first masking tape made from cellulose. It was originally used in auto body shops to paint two-tone cars evenly. People soon began finding other uses for it. The original cellulose tapes were biodegradable, but during World War II tape manufacturers started to use synthetic resins, and now the majority of today's tape (aside from those listed above) is mixed with synthetic resins that never biodegrade.

GLUE

Glues date back more than 200,000 years, to when Neanderthals used tar from birch bark to fix their tools. The ancient Egyptians, Greeks, and Romans also made glue by boiling animal bones, fat, and skin. The Egyptians used glue sparingly since it was expensive, reserving it for the Pharaohs' tomb furniture and to reinforce papyrus scrolls.

You can make your own two-ingredient glue perfect for use in arts and crafts like découpage, papier-mâché figures, or a piñata. Pour ½ cup (70 g) all-purpose flour into a medium-size bowl. Add ¼ cup (60 ml) warm water and mix. Continue to stir until the mixture is thoroughly combined. If you feel it's too thick, add 1 to 2 more tablespoons of water. Transfer the contents to a sealable glass jar and store in the fridge. If the mixture dries up, just add warm water and stir again.

FACT White glue, also known as wood glue or school glue, is a synthetic thermoplastic emulsion of polyvinyl acetate (PVA; RIC #7), water for consistency, and other substances like ethanol to keep the compound from drying out.

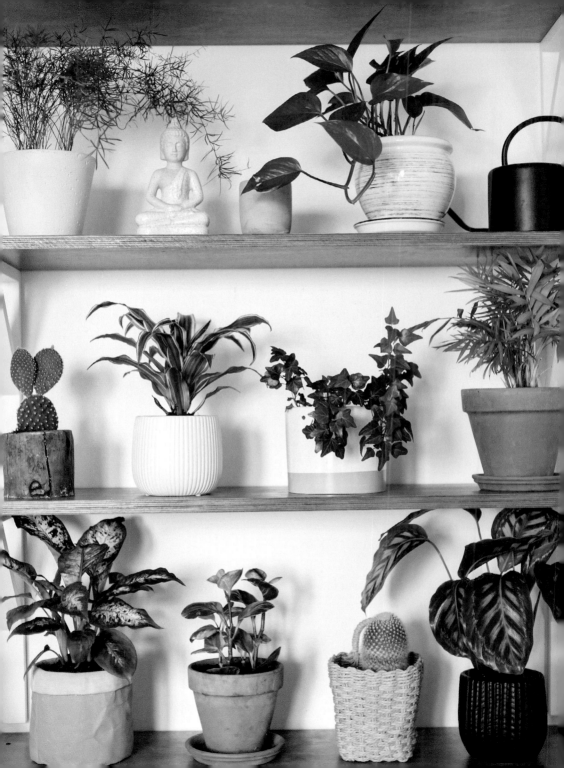

GARDENING POTS

Instead of buying plants in plastic pots, look for varieties in terra-cotta or ceramic pots. As for the plastic pots you already own, first reuse them as long as possible and then recycle them at a garden center like the Home Depot, since not all curbside recycling centers accept these pots. Some farmers' market stands that sell seedlings will reuse the trays and pots when you return them.

When shopping at a garden center, look for sturdy wooden or metal gardening tools and watering cans.

FACT Every year in the United Kingdom, an estimated 500 million plant pots and seed trays are sold and then tossed within a year of purchasing. In the United States, an estimated 350 million tons of plastic—the equivalent weight of twenty-two space shuttles—are produced in the gardening business every year.

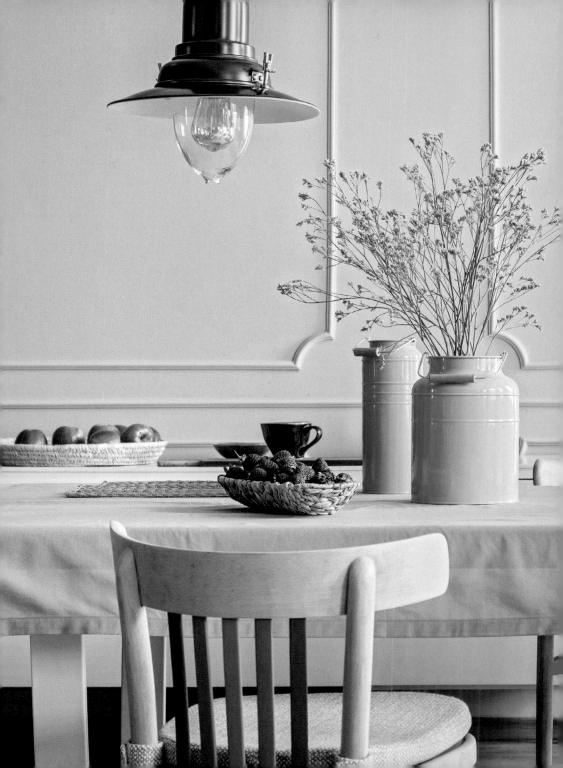

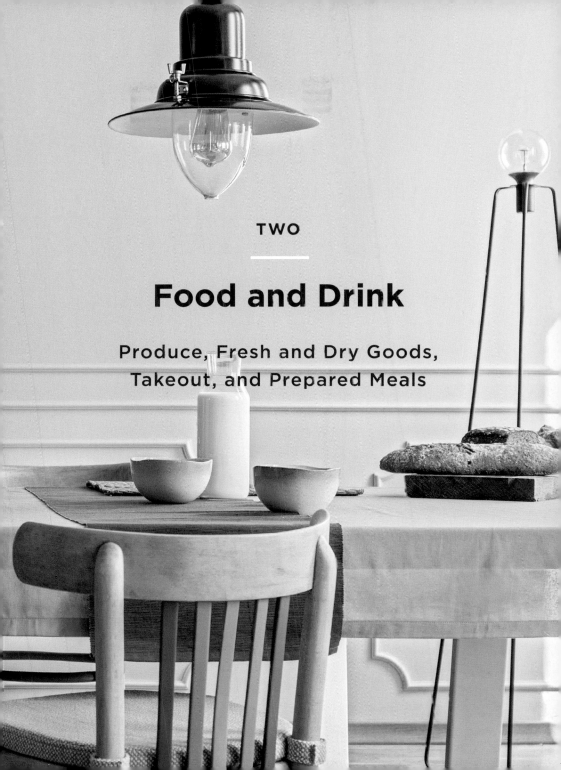

TWO

Food and Drink

Produce, Fresh and Dry Goods,
Takeout, and Prepared Meals

With aisles and aisles of products packaged in plastic at the supermarket, you may be dismayed by the lack of choices for items that are free from bags, clamshells, and wrappers. Ordering food for delivery is just as discouraging, as it usually arrives in plastic bags filled with plastic containers, utensils, and condiments in plastic packaging. However, there are alternatives when shopping for food and ordering takeout.

Whether you eat at home or on the go, your meal is bound to involve items of plastic, most of which are designed to be used just once. Of the 448 million tons of plastic produced in 2015, half of it was made for single-use products. At your typical beach cleanup, 70 percent of the items found polluting the oceans and its shores are food- and beverage-related packaging: bottles and bottle caps, wrappers and containers, straws and stirrers, bags, cups, plates, and utensils.

This chapter explores ways to purchase, prepare, and consume food and drinks by creating your own convenience—without all the plastic packaging.

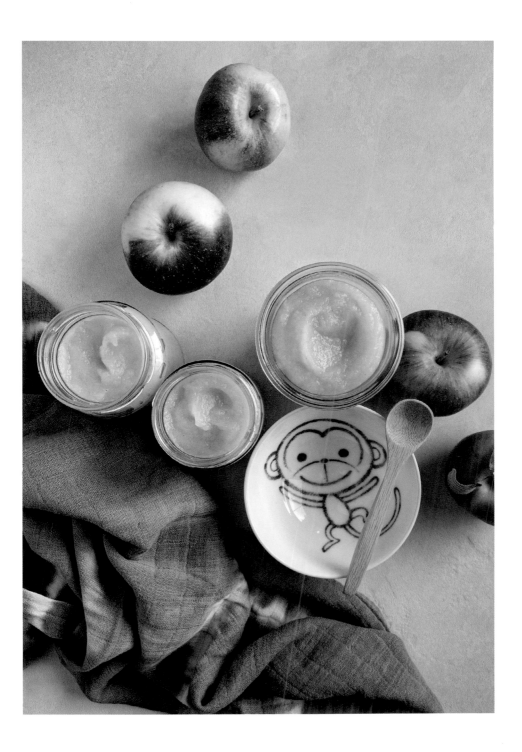

BABY FOOD AND DRINKS

Feed your child real food instead of what you find in convenience pouches. Make your own applesauce and other baby foods by steaming batches of fruits and vegetables until softened. Let them cool before blending. Portion the purée into a stainless-steel ice cube tray and freeze for at least four hours. When frozen solid, transfer these cubes into glass jars and store in the freezer. Using real ingredients creates a good foundation for a healthy, nutritious diet and introduces your child to foods that you eat.

Skip the sugary juices and opt for water in a reusable bottle. To add some flavor, include fruit, such as strawberries, oranges, or cucumber slices.

FACT Invented in 1962, the doypack, commonly recognized as the juice pouch or stand-up pouch, is made of a multilayering of plastic, paper, and aluminum. To recycle them, a special machine is required to separate and process the materials. As a result, only 2 percent of these pouches get recycled, which means 1.4 billion juice pouches end up in landfills every year.

DRINKS

Skip the plastic bottles, artificial ingredients, and excess sugar found in soft drinks by choosing better options. Drink water infused with fresh produce like sliced berries, citrus or tropical fruits, cucumber, or mint if you crave a little flavor. Infused water not only tastes great, it also gives your beverage added nutrients. Refill your bottle several times or drink up and then snack on the fruit. If you crave a fizzy drink, add carbonation using a SodaStream soda maker or a classic glass soda siphon (see Resources, page 237).

If you must purchase a soft drink, choose returnable glass bottles or aluminum cans when possible, and be sure to recycle them.

> **FACT** Americans drink an average of 44 gallons (167 L) of soft drinks per person every year, more than any other country in the world. That's the equivalent of every man, woman, and child drinking 286 bottles. Mexico ranks second at 39 gallons (148 L) and Chile third at 33 gallons (125 L).

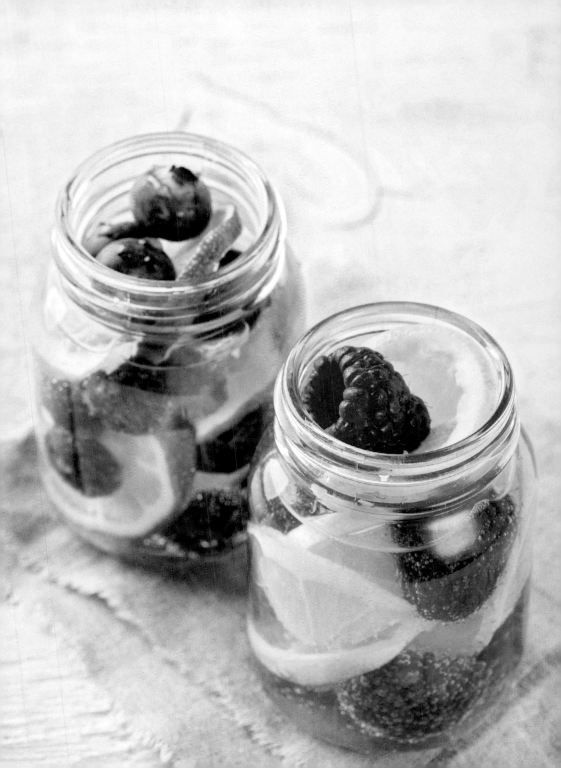

COFFEE

Make your morning brew at home using a French press, a stove-top coffee maker, or refillable pods. For an additional invigorating pick-me-up, repurpose those used (and cooled) coffee grounds into a body scrub with the addition of a little warm water or coconut oil.

When outside your home, either choose your coffee to stay in a café, where it'll likely be served in a good old ceramic coffee mug, or bring your own insulated glass, ceramic, or stainless-steel mug with you—you might even get a discount!

And here's a tip to skip the plastic stirrer: pour the milk and sugar into your coffee cup first, then add the coffee. This will help naturally mix the ingredients for you. Otherwise use a spoon or wooden stirrer.

> **FACT** Fan of those single-use coffee pods? The number of K-Cups in landfills could wrap around the planet 10.5 times. But don't despair: There are plenty of pods that you can refill and reuse (see Resources, page 236).

TEA

Before purchasing tea bags, read the packaging label or contact the brand to see if the bags are biodegradable and compostable, or try composting them at home to see if they break down. Several quality tea brands, including Teapigs and Pukka, use plastic-free tea bags made from cornstarch.

Or just hang loose and opt for loose-leaf tea, which you can steep in a reusable metal tea strainer, or steep fresh herbs in hot water for fifteen minutes to make an herbal tea.

FACT Ninety-six percent of tea brands use bags made from synthetic fibers containing polypropylene, a synthetic resin that seals and is also woven into the paper to help the tea bag retain its shape in boiling water. And the fancier, pyramid-shaped "silky" tea bags are made of nylon which, when heated, leaches phthalates into your cup.

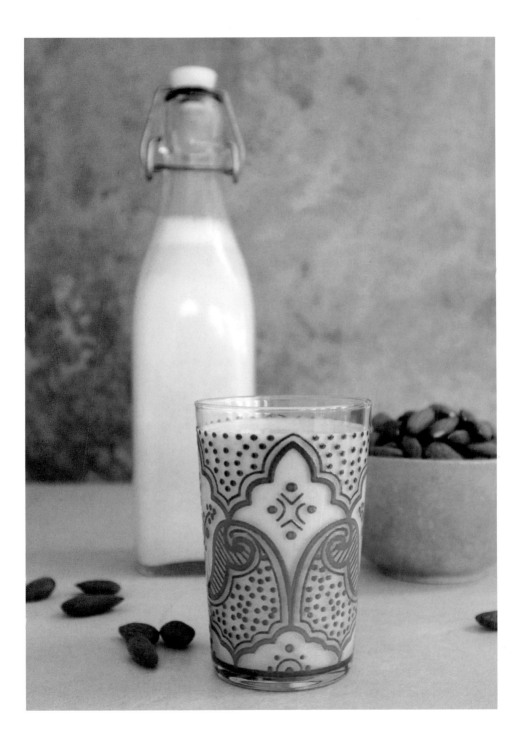

NUT AND SEED MILKS

Skip the packaging by making plant milks at home. It's as easy as blending a few ingredients together.

WHAT YOU'LL NEED

1 cup (140 g) whole raw almonds or cashews

1 tablespoon maple syrup

3 cups (720 ml) filtered water

In a bowl or jar, soak the nuts in water overnight at room temperature.

Drain the nuts and discard the liquid. In a high-speed blender or food processor, blend the soaked nuts with the maple syrup and filtered water. If using almonds, strain the milky blend through a cheesecloth or fine-mesh sieve into a glass jar. (If using cashews, you don't need to strain it.) The milk will last for 3 to 5 days in your fridge.

To utilize the leftover almond pulp, spread a thin layer on a parchment paper-lined tray and freeze it to add to granola or your morning oatmeal. You can also make almond flour by drying out the pulp. Preheat the oven to 200°F (95°C) and spread the pulp out in a thin layer on a parchment paper-lined sheet pan. Bake for 1 to 1½ hours, stirring occasionally, until the crumbs are dry and not clumpy.

Makes 3 cups.

MILK

Bring back the milkman! Not only does milk taste better in glass bottles, it stays fresher and colder, and is sustainable with a bottle-return system. Look for local options at your supermarket, farmers' market, or a nearby farm (see Resources, page 236).

> **FACT** Milk cartons may seem like they're made from paper, but they are coated with a layer of polyethylene to keep them waterproof.

BEER

Avoid the dreaded plastic six-pack rings that animals can get stuck in and choose beer in glass bottles. If you do opt for the aluminum can six-pack, support brands like Heineken UK, that use sustainably sourced 100 percent recyclable and compostable cardboard toppers or check out Saltwater Brewery's biodegradable six-pack rings, which are made from beer byproduct wheat and barley. Just make sure to responsibly recycle those glass bottles and cans.

For a zero-waste option, many craft breweries often offer growler refills.

FACT Six-pack rings, or yokes, are a set of connected LDPE (RIC #4) plastic rings that are commonly used in multipacks of cans. In 1994, the Environmental Protection Agency (EPA) mandated that all ring carriers must be degradable. Rings marked with a diamond symbol are photodegradable and able to break down in three to four months in the light. While this may seem positive, they are often sent to landfills and never degrade.

FRUIT

Many fruits are naturally protected by their peels and skins and there is little need to package them further. If you shop at your local farmers' market, you can bring your own bag or reusable container. The vendors will also happily reuse the containers that portion out their produce.

Pick your own fruits when they are in season. Local farms offer seasonal bounty as well as a fun day out. Consider preserving or freezing some of your harvest for future use (see Resources, page 237).

FACT Stickers on fruits and vegetables are often made of plastic and are neither compostable nor recyclable (because of their small size), and if they make their way down the drain, they contribute to a buildup of trapped material, which can clog the filter of wastewater treatment facilities. In Sweden, at a supermarket chain called ICA, avocados, sweet potatoes, and other produce are labeled "tattooed" by using a low-energy laser to remove the pigment and etch information onto their skins.

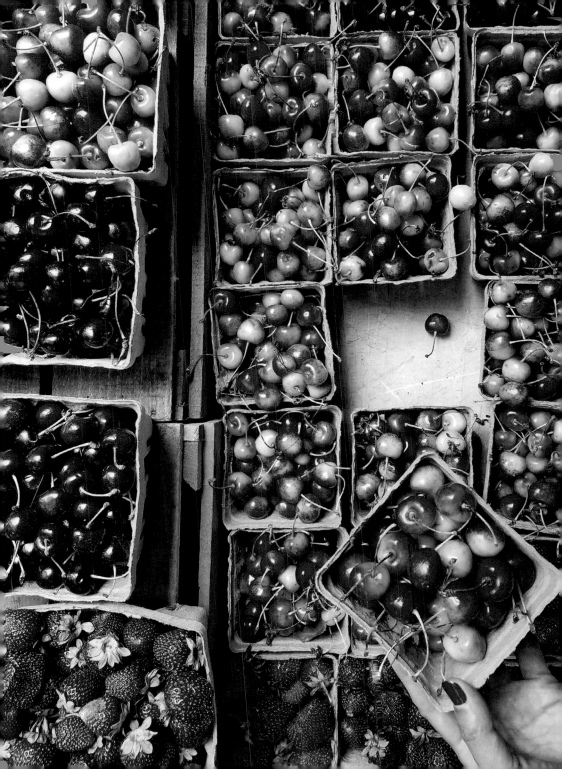

VEGETABLES

Buy "nude" vegetables by shopping at supermarkets, health food stores, food cooperatives, farmers' markets, or international markets, or by participating in community-supported agriculture (CSA), which allows you to enjoy unpackaged, fresh, seasonal bounty. Some companies will even deliver "imperfect" produce with little or no plastic packaging (see Resources, page 236).

When you shop, avoid using the plastic produce bags by bringing your own cloth bags, or use one large tote, if you don't mind your produce mingling (see page 20).

If you buy your groceries online, be sure to include specific instructions like: "Please do not bag in plastic."

FACT While perceived as being more hygienic and keeping foods "fresh," LDPE (RIC #4) packaging can leach chemicals into foods, from prewashed salads in plastic bags to netted bags of loose items like potatoes or Brussels sprouts. It is especially contradictory when you see organic produce wrapped up in plastic! Furthermore, plastic produce bags don't allow for airflow, so if moisture is trapped in the produce, the chances for bacteria growth and spoilage are higher.

MEAT AND SEAFOOD

When meat and seafood are prepackaged, a variety of synthetic material is used—cling film, plastic labels, moisture-wicking pads (made of silica gel, cellulose, and plastic), and Styrofoam trays. To skip the plastic, shop with your own dedicated meat/seafood containers and purchase these items fresh from a butcher or seafood counter in your favorite store or farmers' market. Sanitize the containers for future use with a spray of undiluted white or apple cider vinegar, let it sit for five minutes, wipe clean, and then repeat.

Alternatively, buy from butchers and seafood purveyors who will wrap up your purchases in the traditional way: in wax-lined paper.

FACT Polystyrene is an insulator expanded with air to make Styrofoam. It contains styrene, a chemical compound that the American Cancer Society website lists as "reasonably anticipated to be a human carcinogen." According to the EPA, of the nearly 20 million pounds (9 million kg) of waste that styrene generates annually, about 17.8 million pounds (8 million kg) wind up in the air and 1.7 million pounds (0.8 million kg) get into surface waters.

BREAD

Bread dates back to prehistoric times. The first bread was made from gruel, a porridge-like substance consisting of flour and water. Some say these flatbreads date back thirty thousand years. Ancient Egyptians are credited with the first commercial or widely produced leavened bread thanks to yeast. Keep the bread tradition alive and avoid the plastic packaging altogether by baking your daily bread yourself or buying it from a local bakery. Fresh bread from a bakery usually comes unsliced in a paper bag, which helps it maintain a crisp crust, and most bakeries would also be happy to put a fresh loaf in your own reusable bag.

FACT Plastic packaging aside, there could actually be plastic in the bread you're eating! According to the Environmental Working Group, nearly five hundred commercial baked goods contain azodicarbonamide (ADA), the same chemical used to make yoga mats and flip-flops. ADA is known as the chemical foaming agent of choice. When mixed into polymer plastic gel, it creates tiny gas bubbles that are strong, light, and spongy so it makes bread look puffier and last longer.

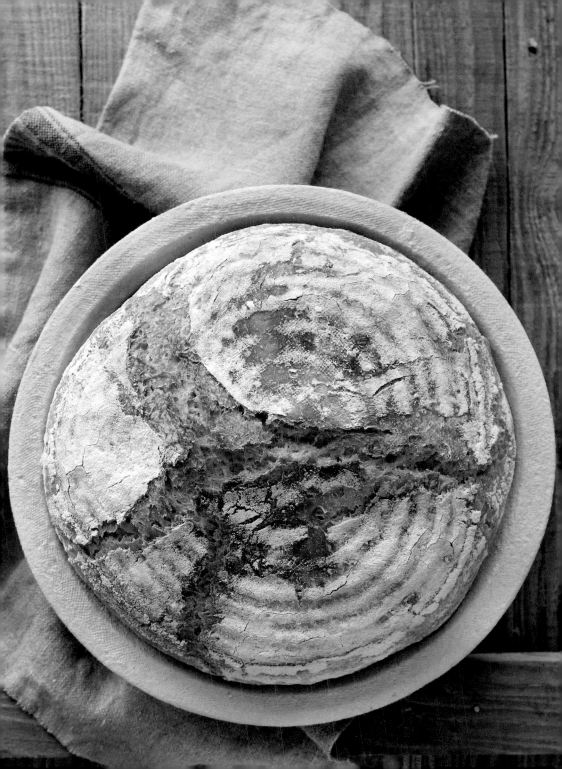

YOGURT

Yogurt is believed to have originated in the sixth century BCE when herdsmen would store their milk in containers made from the stomachs of animals. The result was a tart and thickened milk due to the good bacteria found in an animal's stomach lining. These days a starter culture of living organisms, such as *Lactobacillus bulgaricus*, can be used to make yogurt at home. If you're not quite ready to make your own, opt for purchasing yogurt in refundable glass jars or at least in larger tubs.

FACT The $9 billion yogurt industry in the United States touts the single-serving culture (pun intended). Most yogurt cups are made of polypropylene (PP; RIC #5) plastics. Unless they're repurposed by companies like Preserve, under their Gimme 5 program, most of these cups end up in the landfill, since very few municipalities are able to recycle them.

WHAT YOU'LL NEED

1 quart (32 ounces/950 ml) whole milk

*1 tablespoon fresh, unsweetened store-bought yogurt or yogurt
from a previous batch*

Pour the milk into a Dutch oven and bring to a boil slowly over medium-high heat. Stir occasionally, so the bottom doesn't burn and the milk doesn't boil over.

Once the milk begins to boil, remove the pot from the heat and allow the milk to cool, uncovered, to 110°F (43°C), just warm enough to touch it with a clean fingertip. Stir occasionally to prevent a skin from forming on the surface, but if one does, stir it off and discard.

Gently stir in the yogurt to combine. Cover the pot, wrap it with a blanket or heavy towel, and place it in the oven with the light on. Let it incubate for 9 to 12 hours.

Transfer the yogurt into clean, airtight glass jars and refrigerate. Don't forget to save a couple tablespoons for your next batch.

Makes 4 cups.

ICE CREAM

Skip grocery store ice cream and go to an ice cream shop to have a cone. If you want to keep some at home, ask the server to fill your own container. Alternatively, make your own "nice" cream, using one ingredient: simply slice two bananas and freeze for two hours until firm. In a food processor, blend until smooth and creamy, scraping down the sides of the processor bowl once or twice. Freeze the mixture in an insulated stainless-steel container for one hour, which will help the ice cream stay cold even outside of the freezer.

FACT Store-bought ice cream is packaged in paper coated with plastic, similar to takeout coffee cups and milk cartons.

FROZEN FOODS

Freeze fruits and vegetables when the bounty is in season. Cut corn off the cob, pit and slice fresh peaches, and wash and dry delicious summertime berries. Be sure the berries are completely free of surface moisture before freezing to avoid freezer burn. Spread your prepped fruits and vegetables out on a parchment paper–lined cookie sheet in a single layer to avoid clumping, then stick this in the freezer. Once they are fully frozen, you can store them together in an airtight stainless-steel or glass container. Use the fruits in smoothies or for baking pies, and the frozen vegetables in a stir-fry or soup.

FACT Globus Hypermarket in the Czech Republic has a buy-in-bulk, self-serve selection of frozen fruits and vegetables. Similar to the way you purchase bulk dry goods in supermarkets, you scoop the amount of frozen food you need into a reusable bag.

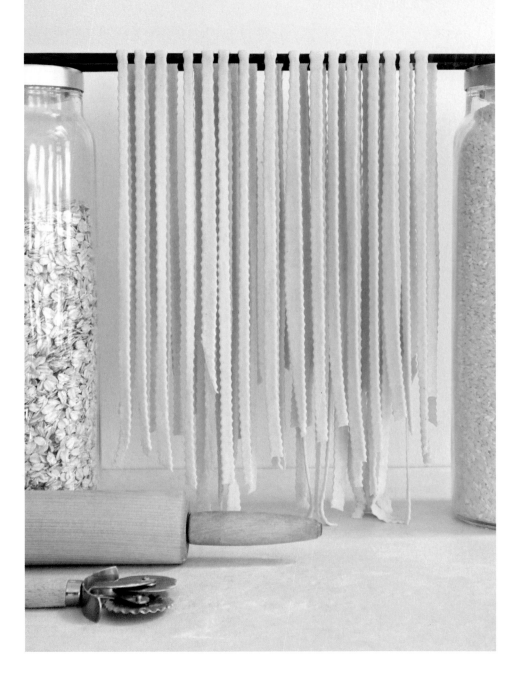

PASTA AND NOODLES

Dry pasta and noodles can be purchased in the bulk sections of some supermarkets, farmers' markets, or restaurants, and you can bring these home using your own containers. Making pasta at home requires only a few ingredients and is an economical option, too.

WHAT YOU'LL NEED

3 cups (420 g) all-purpose flour

1 teaspoon kosher salt, plus more for the pot

1 cup (240 ml) water

2 teaspoons olive oil

In a large bowl, combine the flour and salt. Gradually pour in the water, stirring continuously with a wooden spoon to make a slurry. Add the olive oil and continue to stir until the mixture starts to come together. Knead until a soft ball of dough forms. Continue to knead for 10 minutes, until the dough is smooth and elastic. Let it rest at room temperature, wrapped in a damp dish cloth for 30 minutes.

Bring a large pot of water to a boil. On a clean countertop sprinkled with flour, roll out the dough as thinly as possible and cut out even strips. Boil for 2 to 4 minutes.

Makes 4 servings.

CHEESE

Cheese is alive and needs to breathe, so it shouldn't be wrapped in plastic. To buy the best cheese, visit a deli counter, farmers' market, or specialty cheese shop. Most of these places will wrap your purchases in parchment or cheese paper, or BYO container or beeswax wrap (see page 41).

FACT When wrapped in plastic with no access to oxygen, cheese can produce an ammonia odor or even start to grow harmful bacteria. Because of the high fat and oil content in cheese, the chemicals in plastic wrap are apt to leach onto the cheese.

CONDIMENTS

If you're eating takeout food at home or having a desk lunch at work, keep small bottles of your favorite condiments on hand, and simply refuse to take the packets of ketchup or mustard that are offered in restaurants.

When you order takeout, ask the server to add the condiments directly to your food from the kitchen. If you do want your condiments on the side, ask if they come in a plastic cup or packaging before you accept them.

FACT The innocuous 9-gram packets of condiments (ketchup, mustard, mayonnaise, hot sauce, duck sauce, or soy sauce) that you find in your takeout bag are packed in a nonrecyclable plastic-and-foil package to keep the contents seemingly fresh forever. There isn't an expiration date listed on the sachets themselves (it's listed on the boxes that the packets are delivered in), so there's no knowing how long they've been sitting around. These contents can go "off" quickly, so don't bother collecting a stash. Taco sauce isn't great after four months, while most other condiments expire after eight to nine months.

BREAKFAST CEREAL

If you make your own cereal, you can use whole ingredients and control how much (or how little) sugar you include. Plus, you'll skip the plastic packaging. Recipes for homemade corn flakes, rice cereal, and granola are all within your reach.

Try making the quintessential cornflake cereal on your stove-top. Place an ungreased cast-iron skillet over medium heat. Wait for the skillet to be hot, then pour in 3 tablespoons of water (it should bubble when it hits the pan). Evenly sprinkle 3 tablespoons of finely ground cornmeal and 1 to 2 teaspoons sugar on top of the boiling water across the pan. Without stirring or touching the mixture, let it cook for about 3 minutes until the water evaporates. Flip the pieces over, breaking them into flakes with a bamboo spatula if necessary. Toast for another 3 minutes until crisp. If desired, make another batch and eat immediately.

Makes ½ cup (25g).

> **FACT** Unless your local recycling facility accepts HDPE (RIC #2), cereal box liners are not recyclable.

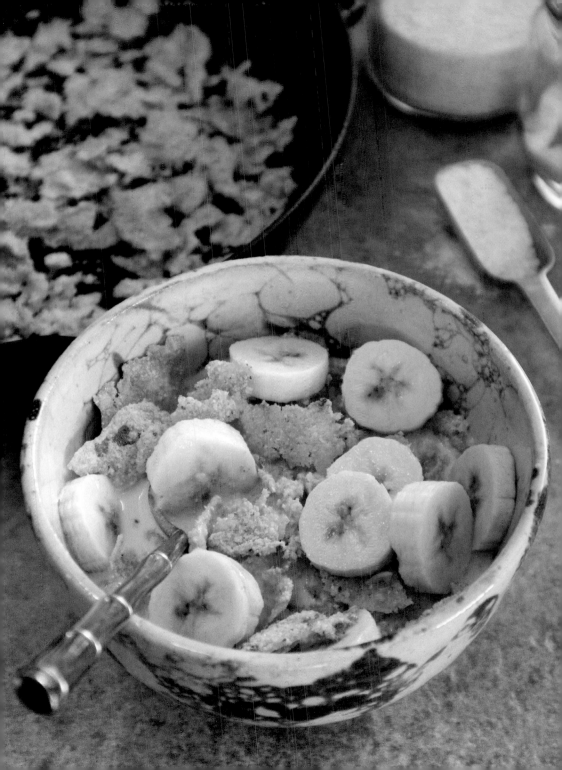

NUTS, SEEDS, AND GRAINS

Most natural food stores and some supermarkets have a dry goods bulk bin section. Always ask the employees if and how you can bring your own containers to avoid using the plastic containers and bags the store provides. Determine the tare (decimal weight in pounds) of your empty glass or stainless-steel jars or sturdy organic cotton bags by placing them on the scale. To avoid confusion at checkout, take a picture of this weight to show the tare of the jar. Type in the PLU (item number) or the price per pound of the food item on this photo and use this for easy checkout. The tare is then deducted from the filled weight of the container. If a store doesn't allow you to use your own containers, a paper bag or a lightweight reusable bag are good solutions. For a list of where to buy in bulk, see Resources, page 236.

Keep in mind that anyone with severe food allergies should not buy ingredients from bulk bins in case of cross-contamination.

TRAIL MIX AND SNACK BARS

Make your own trail mix. It's healthier and more natural than the kinds offered in supermarkets, and it doesn't need any plastic packaging. The ideal trail mix should include 70 percent nuts and seeds for protein (such as cashews, walnuts, pistachios, and sunflower seeds), 20 percent dried fruit for sweetness (raisins, cranberries, apples, or berries), and 10 percent fun stuff (coconut flakes, dried chickpeas, dark chocolate chunks, or sesame sticks). Head to the bulk bin section of your grocery store to pick up these ingredients and mix up a batch. Once you do, you can use the mixture to create your own snack bars.

> **FACT** Pillsbury invented the first plastic-wrapped snack bar, called the Space Food Stick, in the 1960s, which astronauts ate while in space.

continued

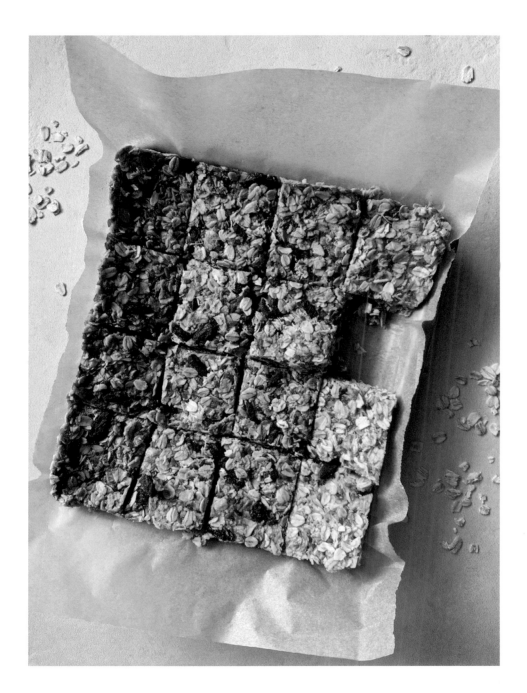

WHAT YOU'LL NEED

1½ cups (180 g) trail mix

1½ cups (150 g) old-fashioned rolled oats

¼ cup (40 g) ground flax seeds

Pinch of salt

½ cup (130 g) nut butter

3 tablespoons honey or maple syrup

2 tablespoons coconut oil

Line an 8 × 8-inch (20 × 20 cm) baking dish with parchment paper.

In a large bowl, combine the trail mix, oats, flax seeds, and salt. Set aside.

In a small saucepan over low heat, melt and mix the nut butter, honey or maple syrup, and coconut oil. Pour this into the dry nut mixture, toss together to combine, and transfer to the prepared baking dish. Press the mixture down firmly in an even layer. Refrigerate for at least 3 hours, then slice into 16 pieces and wrap each with parchment paper or divide into containers for on-the-go snacking. Store in the refrigerator for up to 2 weeks.

Makes 16 snack bars.

SNACKS

Often times our snack choices come wrapped in plastic. Seek out plastic-free options like chocolate-coated nuts, popcorn kernels, and snack mixes in the bulk food bin section in your grocery store, food co-op, or international supermarket. Healthier options include fresh fruit, crunchy vegetables, or a cup of tea.

Next time you go to the movies, skip the plastic popcorn bag by bringing your own popcorn. To make popcorn at home, buy organic kernels from the bulk section of your grocery store.

WHAT YOU'LL NEED

1 tablespoon olive oil

½ cup (100 g) popcorn kernels

Salt

In a medium-size saucepan on high heat, pour enough olive oil to coat the pan, add the kernels, then cover with a tight-fitting lid. Reduce the heat to medium. Shake the pan regularly to prevent the kernels from burning. Once the popping starts, listen until the popping slows to a few pops, take the pan off the burner, and sprinkle with salt to taste. Package in parchment paper bags or reuse a coffee tin for your movie snack.

Makes approximately 13 cups (80 g).

GUM

Did you know most chewing gum has plastic in it? Originally made from chicle (a latex sap from the sapodilla tree native to Central America), chewing gum was popularized during World War II by soldiers. But the chicle supply couldn't keep pace with demand, so scientists learned how to make gum from synthetic rubber and plastic instead of chicle, which also made gum more elastic and less brittle. Opt for all-natural plastic-free gum, like Simply Gum, Chicza, True Gum, or Glee Gum (see Resources, page 237).

> FACT More than 100,000 tons of gum are discarded every year. That's 28,891,233,758 pieces of gum worldwide[1]

SCHOOL LUNCHES AND SNACKS

Look for durable lunch and snack bags made from natural materials, such as organic cotton or wool. For snacks, if you can't give up the zippered bags, silicone snack bags are an option. Stasher Bags, reusable zippered silicone baggies, will upcycle damaged bags into playground pebbles (see Resources, page 237).

Stainless-steel lunch and snack boxes, like ECOlunchbox or PlanetBox (see Resources, page 237), are durable and easy for little hands to use. And for adults, glass jars and wooden bento boxes are great for carrying food around.

FACT Reusable vinyl- and neoprene-lined insulated lunch and snack bags may seem eco-friendly, but through constant use, they tend to degrade, with tiny particles breaking off into your food and the environment.

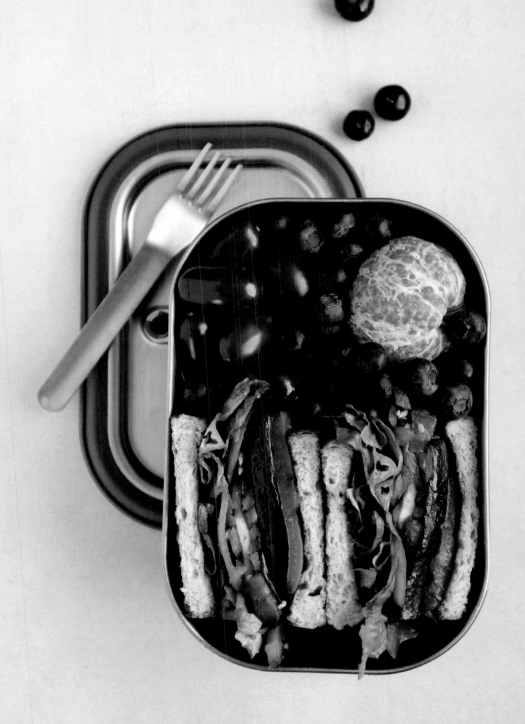

TAKEOUT CONTAINERS

Bring your own washed and sanitized containers to your favorite restaurant for a convenient alternative to plastic takeaway containers. This practice may be greeted with uncertainty because of local health regulations, as some municipalities may restrict restaurants from doing this. An alternative is to ask to be served a plate of food and then transfer it yourself to your own container.

> **FACT** Takeout-related packaging accounts for approximately 269,000 tons of the plastic waste that has entered the oceans. That's equivalent to the weight of twenty-seven Eiffel Towers.

UTENSILS

Be mindful and slip a set of reusable cutlery into your bag. To cut back on carrying numerous reusables, consider carrying a spork (a two-in-one utensil that serves as both a spoon and a fork). If you use disposable bamboo cutlery, be sure to compost it properly.

> **FACT** Americans throw out approximately 40 billion plastic knives, forks, and spoons every year.

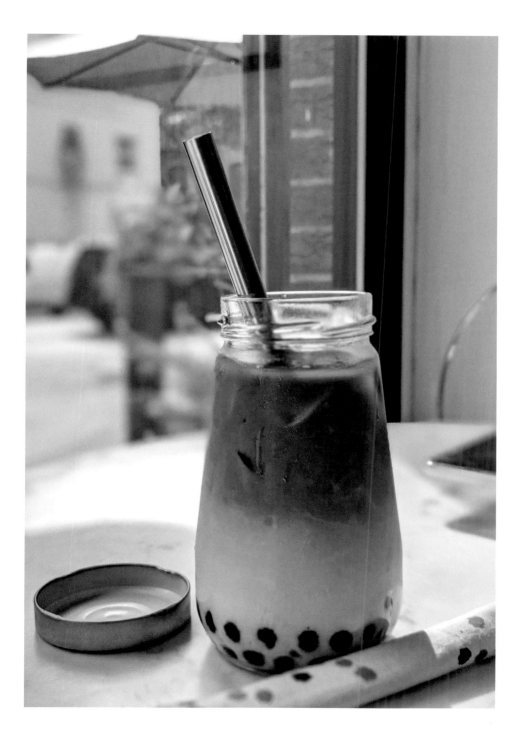

STRAWS

Plastic straws have become one of the leading polluters of our oceans and waterways. Five thousand years ago, Sumerian civilizations used long hollow tubes made from precious metals. Some of the first straws were also simple hollow stems and reeds. In the 1880s, rye grass stalks were used. Wheat stem straws are making a comeback with brands like Hay! Straws and S'wheat, which are 100 percent natural and compostable (see Resources, page 238). For an edible option, try Loliware, which is made from seaweed. You can always skip the sipper or bring your own. Invest in a reusable straw whether it's made of stainless steel, glass, or bamboo. The important thing is to remember to refuse the straw even before a restaurant or bar gives one to you and opt for a paper straw if they have them.

> **FACT** Somewhere between 170 to 390 million straws are used per day in the United States. That's a lot of unrecyclable straws that are only used once and then thrown away.

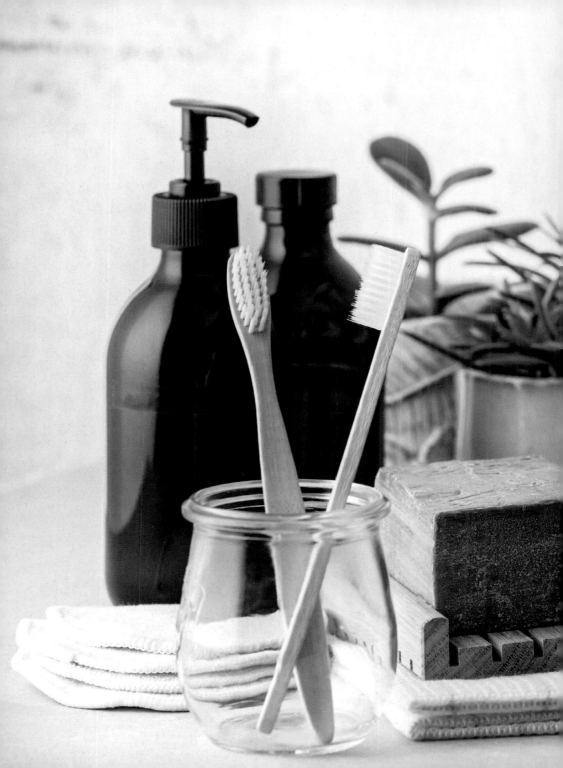

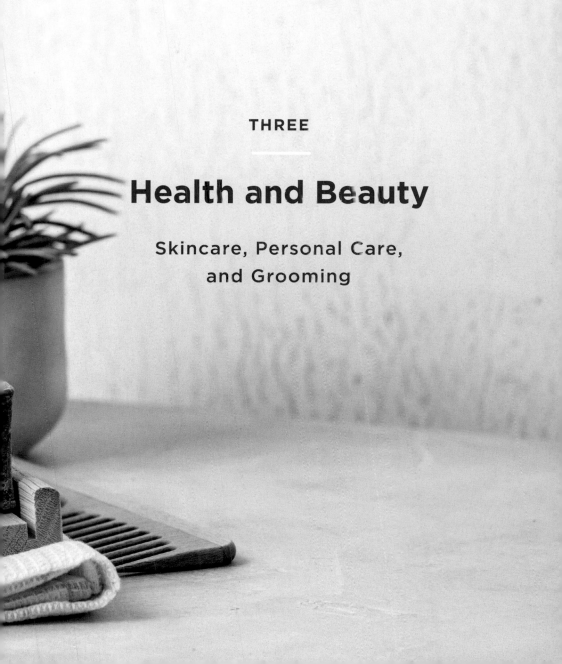

THREE

Health and Beauty

Skincare, Personal Care, and Grooming

In the United States, the average woman uses twelve personal care products daily and the average man uses six. Europeans use an average of seven products per day, and Korean women use an average of thirteen cosmetics a day! Just think of all the plastic tubes, compacts, bottles, and jars sitting in your medicine cabinet or shower—they add up!

In addition to the packaging, plasticizers such as phthalates and other chemicals are added to products to give them different effects and consistencies. From foaming agents in toothpaste to glide-on gel in deodorants, plastic is the culprit. According to the EWG (see page 233), there are anywhere from 85 to 126 unique chemical ingredients in personal care products that we use every day, which are absorbed into our bodies. These chemicals aren't tested to see what long-term effects they have on us. In the United States only 30 chemicals in personal care products have been banned, whereas the European Union and Canada have banned over 1,400 and 600 chemicals, respectively.

But there are ways to keep healthy, fresh, and looking good . . . without the plastic. The solutions in this chapter take into consideration both the packaging and chemical ingredients in the actual product.

MOISTURIZERS

Try making a DIY moisturizer instead of a using store-bought one. An oil-based moisturizer (versus water) works better because it keeps a lot longer.

It also helps to stay hydrated from the inside out by drinking enough water each day. And make sure to use a loofah to exfoliate dead skin (see page 60), which is often mistaken for dry skin.

WHAT YOU'LL NEED

½ cup (140 g) shea butter

2 tablespoons organic coconut oil

2 tablespoons almond oil

Melt the shea butter, coconut oil, and almond oil in the top part of a double boiler, or in a heatproof bowl suspended over a pot of simmering water. Stir the ingredients continuously to melt and mix together, then remove the inner bowl from heat and allow to cool for 30 minutes. When the contents start to solidify, beat the mixture for a minute until it fluffs up. Transfer to lidded glass jars (one for home and a mini one for on the go). Store at room temperature for up to 6 months.

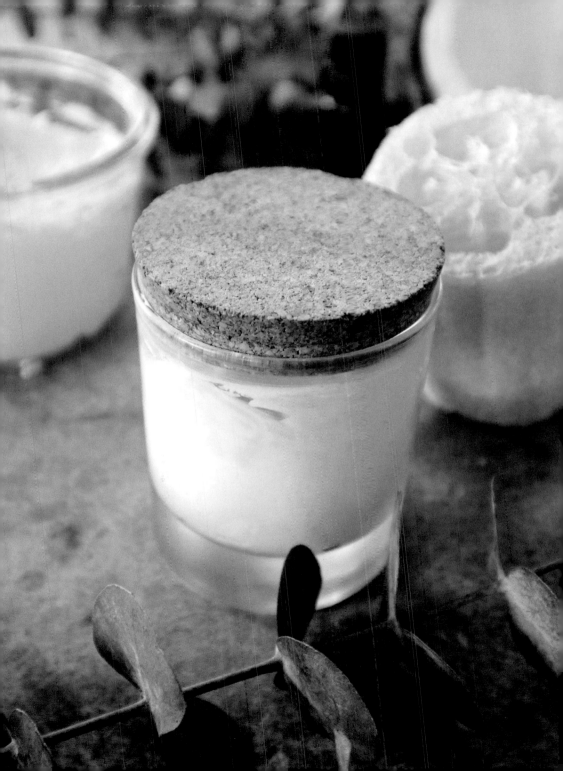

SOAPS

Lather up with bar soap without the packaging. There are plenty of natural, colorful, whimsical options scented with essential oil blends. Try Lush or Soaptopia brands (see Resources, page 238).

> **FACT** Liquid soap in a bottle is often touted as more hygienic than a bar of soap, but studies have debunked this marketing myth. Plus, liquid soap requires about five times more energy to produce than a bar of soap, and it is almost always sold in a plastic bottle.

SHAMPOOS AND CONDITIONERS

Use bar shampoo and conditioner. Some shampoo bars, like African black soap (see Resources, page 233), are good for eighty washes—the equivalent of up to three plastic bottles of liquid shampoo, making them both eco-friendly and cost effective. For an added bonus, there are no airport travel restrictions on bar shampoo. If you want to skip the hair washing, try a DIY dry shampoo. Just lightly sprinkle arrowroot powder or cornstarch onto your roots and rub it in with your fingers or comb through.

For a DIY detangling hair rinse, mix 2 tablespoons apple cider vinegar with 1 cup (240 ml) water in a glass bottle. Be sure to shake the mixture before each use. The mixture helps your hair retain moisture, seals the hair cuticles, and flattens the hair surface, making it easier for you to brush your hair. Always be mindful when using glass bottles in the bathroom so as to avoid breaking them.

FACT Up to 80 percent of shampoo and 95 percent of conditioner is made of water. Considering the global hair care market is worth $88 billion, that's a lot of money on wasted water and plastic packaging. According to Johnson & Johnson, more than 552 million 15-ounce (450 ml) bottles end up in landfills. The number of shampoo bottles thrown out in the United States every year could fill 1,164 football fields.

COMBS AND HAIRBRUSHES

Wooden combs and brushes with bamboo bristles are the simple swaps to get out those tangles without using their plastic counterparts.

FACT In 1878, the comb was one of plastic's earliest applications and replaced the production of combs made from bone, ivory, and tortoiseshell. So ironically, using plastic items once saved elephants and turtles, but now threatens wildlife again.

HAIR GEL AND SPRAY

For centuries people have been using natural mixtures to hold their hair in place. Try your own!

WHAT YOU'LL NEED

2 cups (475 ml) filtered water

¼ cup (40 g) whole brown flax seeds

In a small pot over a medium-high heat, bring the water to a boil. Once it's boiling, pour in the flax seeds, lower the heat, and let the mixture simmer for 10 to 12 minutes, stirring occasionally. You'll know it's ready when the water forms a frothy, gel-like substance. Let it cool down before straining the goopy liquid through a cheesecloth into an airtight glass jar or spray bottle. Store in the refrigerator and use within 2 to 3 weeks or until the mixture starts to get cloudy. You can reuse the seeds or simply add them to your smoothies, granola, or baked goods.

FACT The spray-in-a-can concept was first applied during World War II for insect repellent to protect soldiers from getting malaria. The beauty industry quickly adopted this concept for hairspray. A synthetic water-soluble polymer called polyvinylpyrrolidone is what holds your hair in place.

HAIR TIES

There are many ways to tie long hair with items you already have, such as bandannas, bobby pins, and even a pencil or chopsticks. Or purchase organic cotton and rubber hair ties (See Resources, page 238).

FACT The majority of hair ties are made from plastic or packaged in plastic and have a limited life span because they break easily, get lost, and stretch out quickly. They are also not recyclable.

HAIR COLOR

Color your locks with henna in bar or powder form. Be sure to use natural, reusable rubber gloves when applying the dye. Before applying it to all of your hair, always do a test to a small patch of hair that isn't in plain sight (behind your ear, for example) to be sure you like the color and that you won't have an allergic reaction. Or, embrace your natural hair color, even grays!

FACT In Europe, nearly 60 percent of all women and 10 percent of men use hair dye. In the United States, 75 percent of women and 7 percent of men use it. That translates into roughly 92,000 tons of dye down the drain and into wastewater treatment plants.

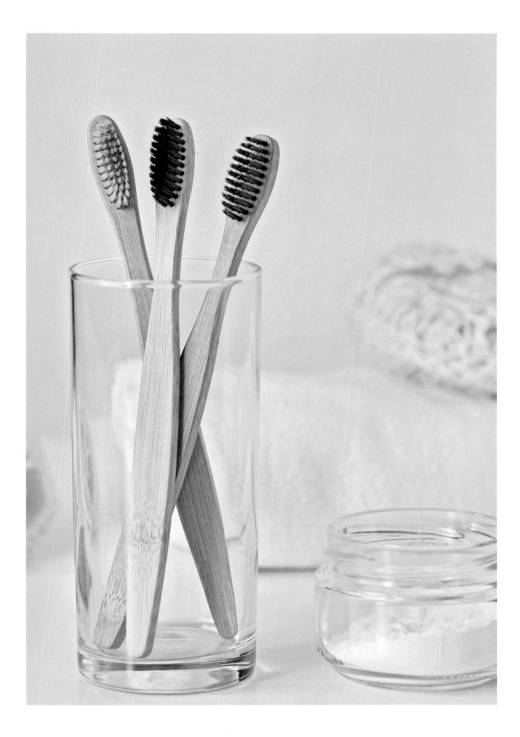

TOOTHBRUSHES

Go retro! The first toothbrushes were made in China in the fifteenth century and they were made of bamboo. Today you can find toothbrushes made with a compostable bamboo handle and partial plant-based bristles mixed with nylon (which should be removed before properly composting the bamboo handle). Or reuse the toothbrush to clean things like your shoes or tile grout. Currently the only alternative to nylon bristles are those made from boar hair.

FACT Each of us will replace at least 300 toothbrushes during our lifetime—that's the equivalent of 12 pounds (5.5 kg) of landfill waste. Now imagine multiplying that by 327 million (the population of the United States). That's 98 billion toothbrushes, or 3.9 billion pounds (1.7 million kg) of plastic, the equivalent of seventy Statues of Liberty.

TOOTHPASTE

Brush those pearly whites with homemade tooth powder! In a small airtight glass jar, combine 2 tablespoons baking soda with ⅛ teaspoon fine sea salt and 1 tablespoon melted coconut oil. Add 1 to 3 drops of peppermint, spearmint, or cinnamon essential oil for flavor. You can also add glycerin-free stevia to cut out the saltiness of the baking soda and salt, if you prefer a sweeter taste. Use a small spoon or sprinkle the powder on your toothbrush. This toothpaste will last about two weeks.

FACT Every year, more than 400 million toothpaste tubes are thrown away in the United States, and 1 billion worldwide. The majority of tubes can't be recycled because they are made from mixed materials, such as aluminum, plastic, and nylon.

DENTAL FLOSS

Seek out 100 percent silk dental floss (see Resources, page 239). It is coated in a natural wax and comes in a refillable glass jar instead of a plastic dispenser. Strong cotton thread lightly coated with coconut oil is also a good DIY option.

FACT If everyone in the United States were to floss their teeth according to the American Dental Association's recommendations, in a year's time the empty containers would fill a hole the size of a football field that's six stories deep.

MOUTHWASH

For a breath-freshening beverage, drink mint or fennel tea or water infused with a cinnamon stick. You can also chew on some fresh parsley to improve your breath after a particularly garlicky meal. Or make your own mouthwash and store it in a decorative glass bottle to beautify your bathroom and freshen your breath.

WHAT YOU'LL NEED

1 cup (240 ml) filtered water

8 drops of peppermint or spearmint essential oil, safe for internal use

2 to 3 drops of liquid stevia (optional)

Combine the water and essential oil in a bottle. Add a few drops of liquid stevia for sweetness, if desired. The mixture keeps for a few weeks at room temperature, or for several months if refrigerated. Pour some into a travel-size glass spray bottle for an on-the-go breath freshener.

FACT Most commercial brands of mouthwash are packaged in plastic bottles and, like toothpaste, contain toxic ingredients that are tough on the environment and your body. Read the warning label on the bottle in case it's accidentally swallowed.

DEODORANTS

You can make your own deodorant. Baking soda neutralizes odors, cornstarch absorbs moisture, and tea tree oil has antibacterial properties to keep odors at bay. Reuse an empty, clean spice jar to store the mixture, and avoid the chemicals and the plastic packaging of a commercial brand.

WHAT YOU'LL NEED

2 tablespoons aluminum-free baking soda

2 tablespoons cornstarch

2 to 3 drops of tea tree oil

Fill a glass jar with all the ingredients, cover, and shake to combine. Sprinkle a little onto your hands and apply to your armpits.

FACT Did you know the first commercially produced deodorant didn't make its debut until 1912? It became widely adopted thanks to an aggressive marketing scheme. The reality is that not everyone sweats or smells badly when they do. It all boils down to your cleanliness, genes, and diet.

RAZORS

Switch to a safety razor made entirely from metal with a replaceable blade. Albatross Designs is one maker of safety razors (see Resources, page 239) dedicated to curbing plastic pollution, and will take back your used blades. Alternatively, try sugaring or other plastic-free waxing options (see Resources, page 239).

Did you know that on average, women pay 11 percent more for razors and razor cartridges than men do? Reusables are typically unisex, so if you're a woman, purchase these and you'll be able to avoid the "pink" tax.

SHAVING CREAMS

Try a brush made from natural bristles and an old-school shave soap, adding water to build up the lather. A bar of shaving soap will last a lot longer than shaving cream in a can and is virtually package free.

FACT Shaving cream in a can is prelathered, meaning that water has already been added. In other words, you are paying extra for water and getting less product.

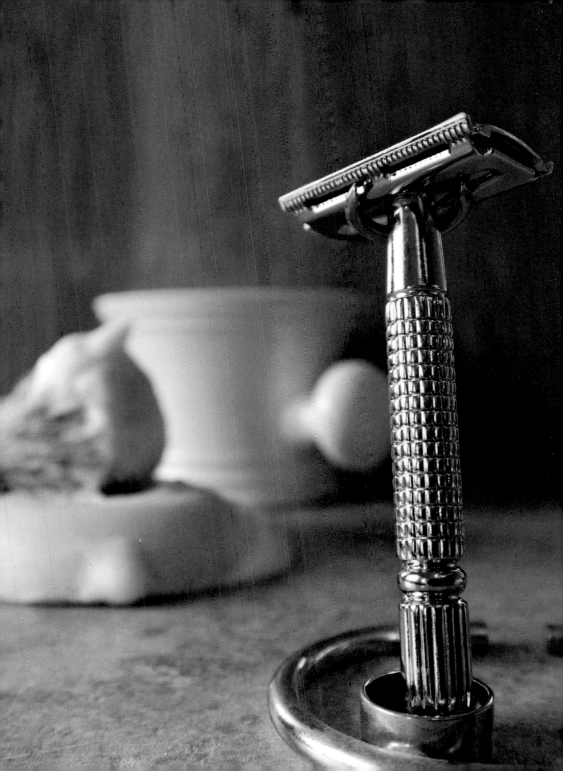

COSMETICS

Instead of covering up your physical beauty, let your face glow naturally. Start with maintaining a daily routine that includes a healthy diet, exercise, a good night's sleep, and lots of water to help you look beautiful without makeup. You can also opt for minimally packaged cosmetics or those sold in cardboard, glass, wood, metal, or tin packaging. Some brands also offer refills (see Resources, page 239).

As you start to phase out plastic from your daily skincare and cosmetics, Origins store locations will accept and recycle your empty plastic cosmetic containers regardless of the brand (see Resources, page 239).

FACT Throughout history, from ancient Egypt to the Renaissance, men and women used cosmetics for protection from the sun, as an indication of class, or for conventions of beauty. Made from common ingredients, these cosmetics were stored in boxes or reusable vessels. Nowadays, the beauty industry produces 142 billion units of disposable plastic packaging worldwide, including containers for foundation, concealer, lipstick, lip gloss, lip balm, mascara, eye shadow, eyeliner, eyebrow gels, blush, powder, bronzer, nail polish, and the list goes on.

MAKEUP REMOVERS

Keep it simple! Only one ingredient is needed for the job—organic coconut oil, the kind that comes in in a glass jar. Apply it with a reusable cotton square (see page 146). Coconut oil also doubles as an overnight moisturizer once you've cleaned your face.

FACT Makeup wipes are made from a combination of things like cotton, wood, pulp, and plastic fibers (polyester and propylene). When they get flushed down the toilet, they wreak havoc on the sewage system because they create buildups that need to be removed manually.

COTTON SQUARES

You can make your own cotton pads from cloth made from natural fibers, such as organic cotton flannel or bamboo.

WHAT YOU'LL NEED

½ yard (45 cm) organic cotton flannel or bamboo fabric

Needle and thread

Prewash the fabric and cut it into 2- or 3-inch squares instead of rounds (to avoid leftover fabric scraps). Sew 2 pieces together with a blanket stitch so the edges don't fray. Store your cotton squares in a glass jar or stainless-steel container. After use, rinse by hand and allow to air-dry to be ready for the next use.

FACT Commercial cotton squares or rounds are often blended with plastic fibers (rayon and viscose), bleached, and treated with pesticides. Plus, they also always come in a plastic bag.

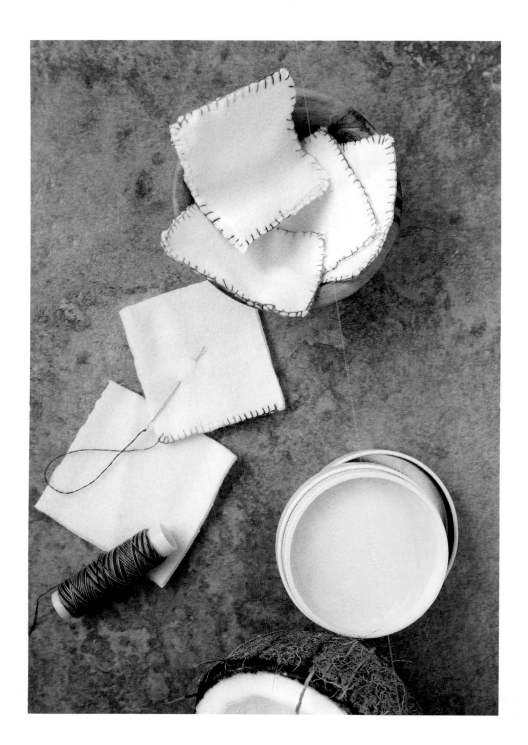

COTTON SWABS

If you must use a cotton swab to clean your ears, use plastic-free or reusable cotton buds or a bamboo ear pick/ear curette, which is commonly used in Asia (see Resources, page 239).

> FACT Some Q-tips (originally known as quality tip) are made with plastic sticks. These often get flushed down the toilet, pass through water treatment plants, and end up in the ocean.

TOILET PAPER

Look for rolls that are made of 100 percent bamboo or recycled and unbleached paper that aren't packaged in plastic film. Who Gives a Crap toilet paper is made from 100 percent recycled paper, with 50 percent of profits going to help build toilets for those in need in Asia, Africa, and Latin America. If you have a bidet in your bathroom, you can forgo the toilet paper altogether.

FACT Toilet paper rolls are typically bunched together in a plastic film. Much like the plastic grocery bag, this film is not accepted at all recycling facilities because it can get stuck in the gears of the machinery.

HANDKERCHIEFS

Skip the tissues and keep it clean with organic cotton hand-kerchiefs just like the ones your great-grandfather used to use. You can repurpose an old T-shirt, pillowcase, or sheet to make them yourself. When on the go, store clean handkerchiefs in a small bag or pouch and have a separate bag for soiled ones. The used hand-kerchiefs can be cleaned with your whites in a hot wash.

FACT The tissue as we know it was first introduced in 1924 and marketed as a way for ladies to remove their cold cream. By the 1930s, Kleenex pivoted directions and began marketing tissues for runny noses with the slogan "Keep that cold to yourself." Believe it or not, snotty tissues are not recyclable, and Americans use upward of 255 billion disposable facial tissues a year!

FEMININE CARE

Reusable menstrual cups, pads, and period panties make it easy to be waste-free while also saving money in the long run. A menstrual cup can cost anywhere from $20 to $40 but can last up to four years or more, which compared to tampons would represent a savings of up to $460 over those four years.

FACT The average menstruating woman uses 250 to 300 pounds (110 to 135 kg) of pads, tampons, and applicators in her lifetime. These all contain plastic, and since they're combined with human waste, they must be sent to landfills. Or, even worse, tampons and applicators are flushed down the toilet, where they wreak havoc on sewage systems and can pollute our oceans.

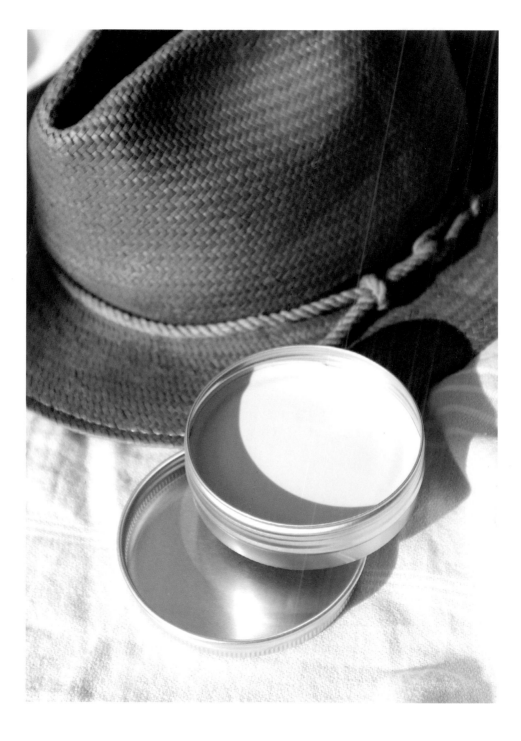

SUNSCREENS

Most sunscreens are made with chemical filters that are then absorbed through the skin. The safest bet is to choose mineral-based sunscreens such as zinc oxide and titanium dioxide and find one packaged in a tin (see Resources, page 240).

> **FACT** An estimated 14,000 tons of sunscreen lotion wind up in the oceans every year. Scientists have discovered that sunscreens with oxybenzone and octinoxate contribute to the bleaching of coral reefs.

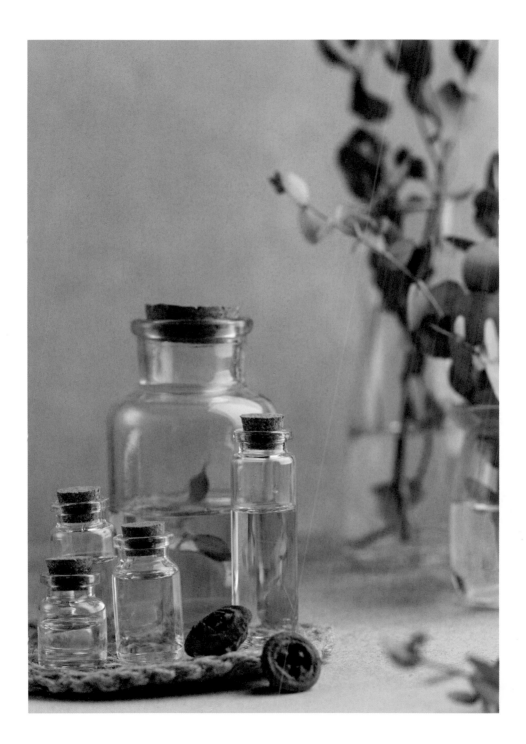

INSECT REPELLENTS

Buy repellent in a tin or a glass bottle (see Resources, page 240). For more natural alternatives in spray, look for eucalyptus oil, which has been acknowledged by the Centers for Disease Control (CDC) to be an effective repellent. If you want to skip the spray, use a burner to diffuse essential oil of citronella, or light citronella candles on summer evenings. Some people find that eating plenty of garlic or chili peppers keeps the mosquitoes away. Minimize the amount of skin exposed by wearing long-sleeved shirts, pants, and knee-high socks.

FACT Diethyltoluamide (DEET), the most common ingredient in insect repellents, is a chemical that deters insects with its strong smell. DEET is also a solvent that can melt some plastic (though not the bottle it's packaged in)—so if you use it and suddenly find a hole in your shirt, you'll know why.

BANDAGES

Scrapes and boo-boos don't need to be covered up with toxic chemicals. Our skin has an incredible power to heal on its own. First clean the wound with natural soap and water. For a wound that needs protection, try a Patch strip (see Resources, page 240), a bamboo adhesive or an organic cotton gauze bandage secured with a knot or paper medical tape, which is better for you, your child, and the planet. A kiss to make it better goes a long way, too.

FACT Historically, wounds were covered with mixtures of substances including mud or clay, plants, and herbs to heal. Nowadays we tend to use chemical ointments, plastic strips, and even polymer compounds (liquid bandages). Bandages are commonly made from polyvinyl chloride, polyethylene, or polyurethane and a latex woven "fabric." Not only are these bandages not degradable, the chemicals can get absorbed into the open wound.

EARPLUGS

Opt for natural beeswax earplugs. They're easy on the ears and on the planet, as they're made from a biodegradable material.

FACT Using beeswax as a sound barrier is a tried and tested method used throughout the centuries. In Homer's classic tale *The Odyssey*, written in the eighth century BCE, the goddess Circe warns Odysseus to wear earplugs made of beeswax when sailing by the Sirens who lured sailors to their death with sweet songs.

CONTACT LENSES

If glasses and Lasik aren't for you, stick with two-week or monthly contact lenses instead of daily disposable ones. And don't flush your old contacts down the toilet or sink! Recycle them along with the blister packs and foils through the Bausch + Lomb and TerraCycle "One by One Recycling Program" (see Resources, page 240).

FACT Contact lenses are made of a soft plastic material that absorbs water. In the United States, more than 45 million people wear contact lenses, throwing away 14 billion lenses a year, which is equivalent to 441,000 pounds (200,000 kg) of plastic. Approximately 15 to 20 percent of these contacts are thrown down the toilet or sink, finding their way to water treatment plants, where they become part of the agricultural sludge used by farms for their soil, polluting the earth and entering the food chain.

CONTACT LENS SOLUTION

For hygienic reasons, there are no DIY or refillable bottle schemes for contact lens solution. After all, the eyes are one of our most sensitive organs, and cleanliness is key. The good news is you can recycle the lens solution bottles.

First, see if your curbside recycling will accept your solution bottle by looking for the Resin Identification Code (RIC) or number with chasing arrow (see page 16) typically found on the bottom of the bottle. Many bottles are made from polyethylene terephthalate (PET; RIC #1), which is accepted by most curbside recycling programs. If not, try the TerraCycle "One by One Recycling Program" (see Resources, page 240), just don't include the cardboard box.

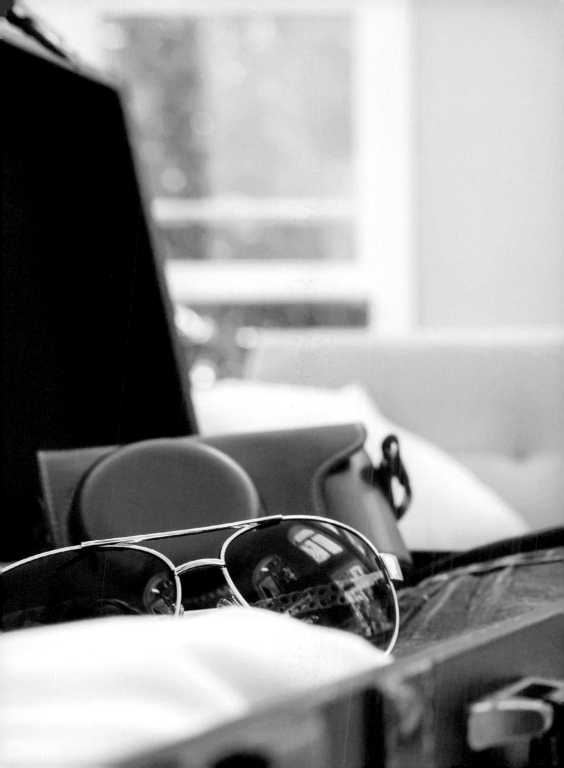

FOUR

On The Go

Travel, Business, and
the Great Outdoors

Often incorrectly touted as disposable, single-use plastics are especially pervasive while on the go because of their light-weight convenience. But spending more time outside of the home—whether at work, at school, or traveling—doesn't mean we have to increase the amount of plastic we use. There are solutions.

In the United States, the concept of disposability is connected to the surge in plastic production shortly after World War II. Initially, in the 1950s, people were so accustomed to reusing beverage bottles or coffee cups that advertising companies had to teach them to trash items after one use. The throw-away culture was quickly adopted. The world's annual plastic production in 1950 was 2.3 million tons. Fifty years later, pro-duction increased a hundred times to 200 million tons.

You don't have to buy into the 1950s hype that skipping plas-tic is tantamount to forgoing convenience while you travel or exercise. This chapter explores a variety of solutions that can lighten your load and plastic footprint while on the go, includ-ing using apps and lightweight reusable materials.

RECEIPTS AND TICKETS

Most receipts are printed on thermal paper, a process that uses heat instead of ink to print text on paper that is coated with BPA, an industrial chemical used in certain plastics. Skip the receipt, opt for an e-receipt, or take a photo of the register screen for your records. If a hard copy is your only option, wash your hands with soap and water as soon as possible to decrease your skin absorbing BPA and definitely don't put the receipt in the bag with your groceries to avoid contaminating food items.

Movie tickets, airline tickets, concert tickets, and boarding passes are also typically printed on thermal paper. If you scratch the printed side of a movie ticket with a coin and a dark mark appears, then it's thermal paper. So go paperless and use a digital ticket. If you need a physical ticket, print it on 100 percent recycled paper. Don't recycle thermal paper because it will contaminate the rest of the paper with BPA.

FACT The harmful effects of BPA were accidentally discovered more than twenty years ago. Scientists conducting a fertility experiment on mice were puzzled by the sudden increase in chromosomally abnormal eggs in the female mice. Turns out BPA was leaching from the plastic cages and water bottles after they were cleaned.

BUSINESS CARDS

Download an app to create a digital business card. Not only is it waste-free, but many apps have a built-in system which makes it easier to organize your contacts within the app. AirDrop and Quick Response (QR) codes are also great ways to digitally exchange contact information. Connect via social media platforms like LinkedIn or scan a nametag on Instagram or share your Snapcode on Snapchat.

Digital cards cost 80 to 100 percent less than paper cards. If you do need to print, though, the most environmentally friendly option is to use 100 percent recycled paper without the laminate, foil stamping, or engraving.

Consider repurposing old paper cards into bookmarks or use the blank sides as mailing labels.

FACT In Japan, the *meishi*, or business card, is a very important part of the culture. An estimated 70 million professionals order at least three batches of cards every year. In the United States, 10 billion business cards are printed every year and 88 percent are thrown out in less than a week after they've been shared.

PHONE CASES

Opt for natural materials such as bamboo, wood, or hemp (see Resources, page 240). Pela Case is a compostable phone case that uses straw fibers, or renewable feedstock, a byproduct of the flax harvest in Canada, which would otherwise be burned down at the end of each season. The Pela Case is a circular design product, meaning it can either be composted at home or sent back to Pela Case to be repurposed into a new case.

SUITCASES

Invest in good-quality suitcases, especially if you travel often. When buying luggage made of plastic, opt for post-consumer recycled plastics. A plastic suitcase made from recycled PET (RIC #1) bottles extends the average useful life of a water bottle from twelve minutes to ten years. Otherwise choose a bag made of a sustainable and durable textile such as hemp.

Got a bag with a broken wheel or zipper? Order the parts online and fix it yourself with any number of online tutorials. You'll save money, extend the life of your suitcase, and feel good about your accomplishment. When you are ready to retire your suitcase, consider using it for storage instead of buying a cardboard box.

FACT The majority of suitcases are made from thermoplastics, flexible plastics that melt when heated and can be formed and reformed. The most popular plastics used in suitcases are polycarbonate, ballistic nylon, cordura, polypropylene, and polyester because they are lightweight, durable, and relatively inexpensive.

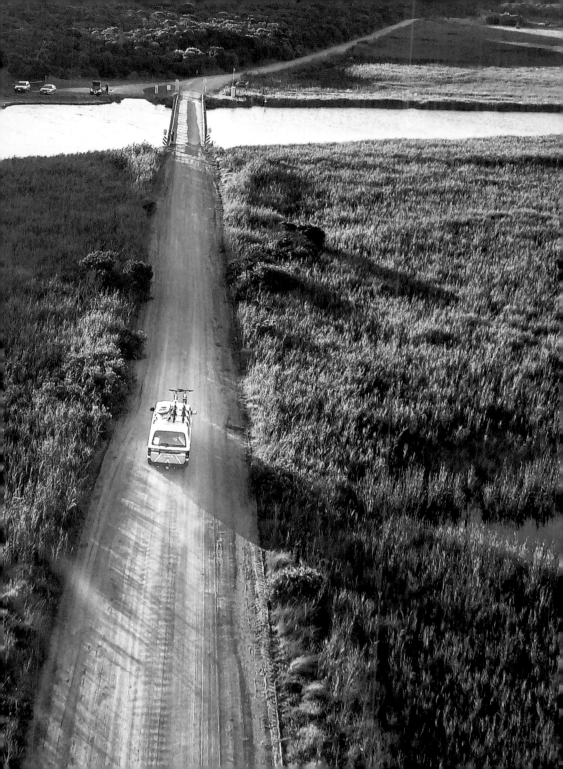

TRAVEL

According to the World Wildlife Fund (WWF), 80 percent of all tourism takes place in coastal areas, with beaches and coral reefs among the most popular destinations. While your efforts to reduce plastic in your daily life protects these destinations, your journey to get there can also be a threat to the environment. So consider driving instead of flying with your family or friends to your next destination. A family of four in a car cuts their carbon footprint in half when compared to flying.

Support eco-friendly destinations, accommodations, and businesses. For example, look for LEED (Leadership in Energy and Environmental Design) hotels, since that certification means the hotel is reducing the property's carbon footprint (see Resources, page 240). Visiting national parks is also a great way to connect with nature and appreciate why your plastic-reducing efforts matter.

HOTEL MINI BAR

Refuse the mini bar in your hotel room and venture out to a local restaurant or supermarket. As convenient as those bottles are, the markup on mini bar items is three to four times the retail price.

Some hotels provide refill stations for your water bottle, or just ask the hotel bar or restaurant to refill your bottle so you can skip buying bottled water all together.

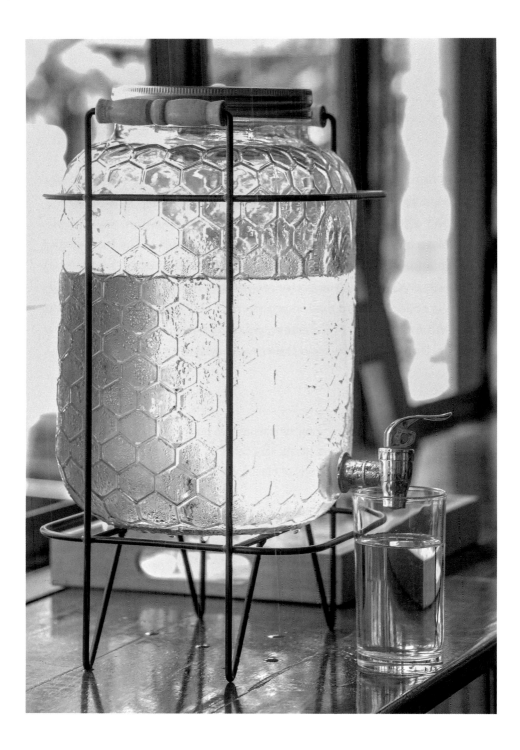

COOLERS

Styrofoam coolers are not so cool. Buy a vintage-style cooler made from steel, aluminum, and chrome, which will surely last long enough to justify the investment. For a lighter but still eco-friendly option, Igloo Recool is made from recycled tree pulp and is economical, reusable, and biodegradable (see Sources, page 249).

FREEZER PACKS

The chemical substance used in a cold pack is called sodium polyacrylate, a superabsorbent polymer also used in diapers and tampons that isn't biodegradable. To make your own cold pack, fill a stainless-steel flask or water bottle with water until three-quarters full (to leave room for expansion). Place the flask in the freezer until frozen. For a lighter cold pack, fill the flask half full with applesauce or another favorite homemade fruit purée, and freeze. Once thawed, this becomes a cool and tasty dessert.

FACT The first chemically made cold pack for food was patented in 1959 and was the precursor for the modern ones. Although the ice packs provided by your meal kit delivery service can be reused, they can't be used indefinitely and will still be destined for a landfill.

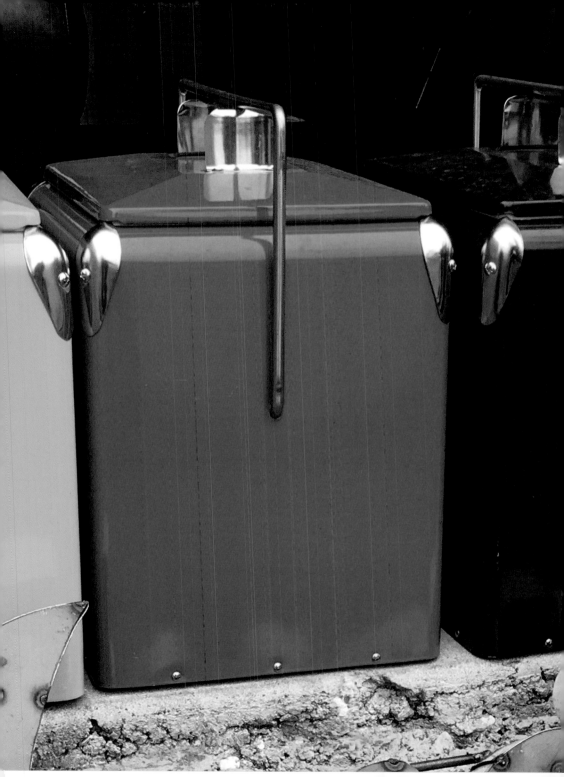

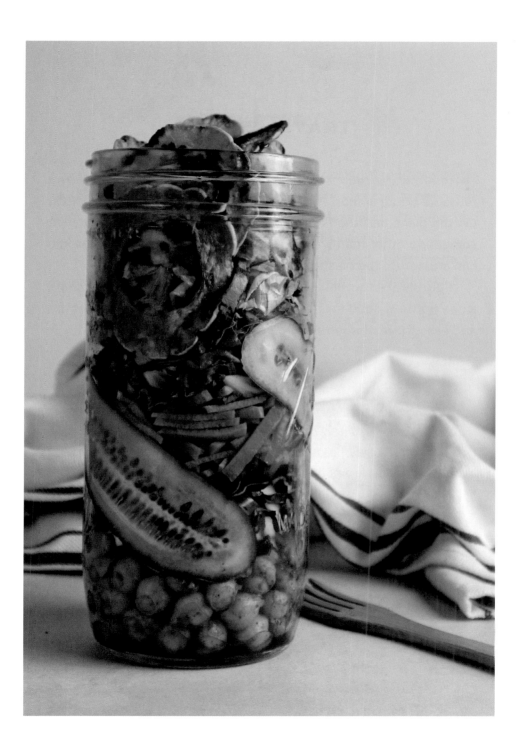

MEALS AND SNACKS ON THE GO

Whether traveling by plane, train, bus, or car, pack food for the trip. Alternatively, make time to sit down and eat at a restaurant before your flight or road trip, rather than opting for grab-and-go meals or buying food at the airport, train station, or rest stop. You'll bypass not only the meal packaged in plastic, but also the cutlery wrapped in plastic film.

FACT Airlines are starting to eliminate different types of plasticware such as straws and cutlery. Others are going the extra mile and getting rid of all single-use plastic.

ATHLETIC SHOES

When you buy new sneakers, do your homework on any company claiming to be eco-friendly and plastic-free. Look for sneakers with materials that are organic and natural. Companies like Veja and Ecoalf use organic materials, including natural rubber or even marine algae instead of plastic soles. While it won't be easy to find completely plastic-free shoes, these companies use post-consumer plastic, even upcycling ocean plastic from fishing nets and bottles. For more guidance on determining which brands are eco-friendly, see Resources (page 241).

FACT Much like athletic clothing, athletic footwear is primarily made of synthetic materials, but that's not the only issue with these shoes. According to an MIT study, a typical carbon footprint to produce a pair of these shoes is 30 pounds (13.5 kg) of carbon dioxide emissions, the equivalent of running a 100-watt lightbulb for one week straight. Two-thirds of its carbon footprint comes from the manufacturing process because the shoes are made in factories powered by coal.

LIGHTERS

Instead of using disposable lighters, buy new or vintage refill-able lighters that will last you a lifetime (see Resources, page 241). These can be refilled with butane gas, which isn't the eco-friendliest choice, but it's better than using plastic disposable lighters. A box of matches will also do the trick.

FACT Studies have shown that in seven years' time, disposable gas lighters and other littered plastics can make their way by certain ocean currents from the shores of the United States all the way to Japan.

YOGA MATS

Buy a natural rubber or cork yoga mat (see Resources, page 241). The upfront cost is more than what you'd pay for a plastic one, but the mat will last a lifetime—and without all of the toxic chemicals.

> **FACT** Most yoga mats contain PVC (RIC #3), a very toxic plastic throughout its life cycle. During the production phase it releases dioxins into the atmosphere. While in use, phthalates used to soften yoga mats are absorbed into the skin or even inhaled through the lungs. When PVC is disposed of in landfills, it will leach harmful chemicals into the soil and water, and if it is incinerated, it will further release harmful dioxins into the air.

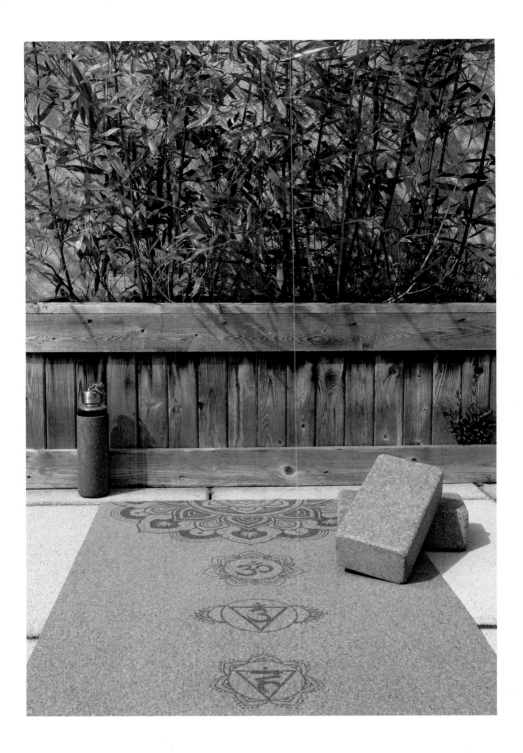

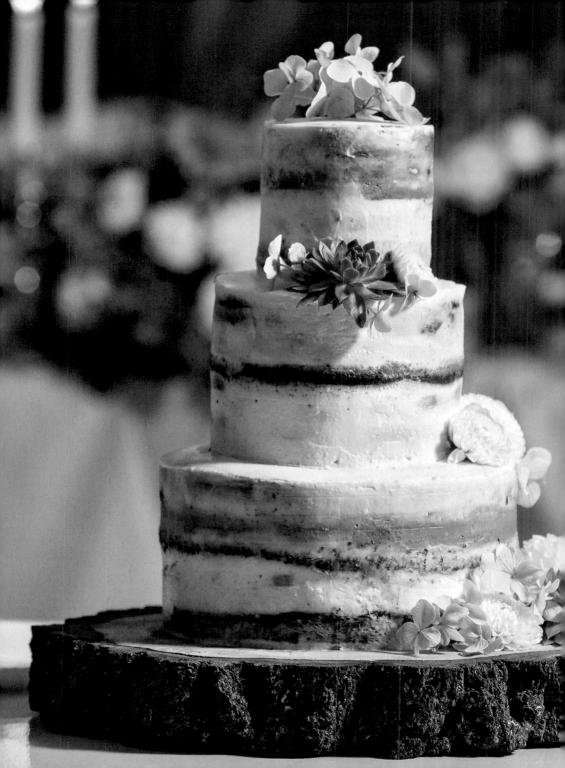

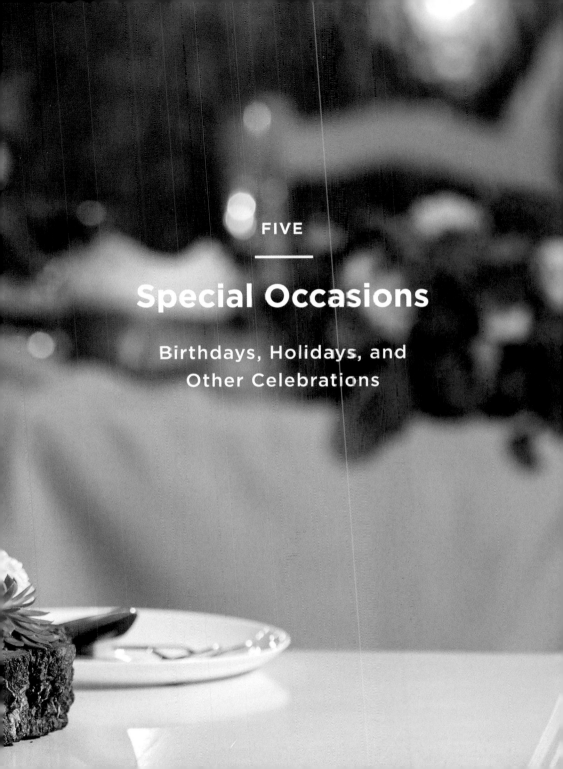

FIVE

Special Occasions

Birthdays, Holidays, and
Other Celebrations

Special occasions such as weddings, birthdays, and holidays that celebrate important life events and traditions don't need to be wasteful and full of plastic. Make your celebrations more about the gathering of loved ones and less about the things we acquire and exchange. This chapter encourages a return to simpler times, when people came together to cook feasts at home with treasured recipes, and decorated with natural materials such as fabric, foods, and elements found in nature. Creating something from scratch doesn't always have to be time-consuming or expensive. Keep it simple. You can reuse or repurpose decorative items. Thanksgiving staples like squash, pumpkin, and cranberries can first be used to create decorative table settings and then transformed into delicious dishes. There are also ways to avoid purchasing manufactured items altogether by buying experiential gifts or sending online gift cards.

PARTY INVITATIONS AND GREETING CARDS

Go paperless! No matter the occasion, there are a variety of online invitation and card options (see Resources, page 241).

For personalized digital invitations and greeting cards, you'll pay a tenth of the price of printed paper ones, or if you keep it simple with predesigned layouts, they can be free. You'll also save on postage and keep your carbon footprint in check.

Need to go the paper route? Print your own invitations and cards on 100 percent recycled paper or get creative and make your own plantable seeded card.

FACT Mylar paper, which is commonly used for wedding invitations, has a metallic and shiny finish that is coated with a plastic film made from Biaxially Oriented Polyethylene Terephthalate (BoPET; RIC #7). This paper is neither recyclable nor biodegradable because of the mixed materials.

WHAT YOU'LL NEED

1 cup (140 g) shredded newspaper or craft paper scraps

1 cup (240 ml) water

1 teaspoon small seeds, such as wildflower, basil, or dill

Dried flowers (optional)

Fine-mesh screen

Place the paper scraps in a blender with water and soak for 15 minutes. Blend until the mixture looks like oatmeal. Drain through a strainer and pat out the excess water.

Transfer the paper pulp to a small bowl and add the seeds. If you want to add a pop of color, sprinkle in some dried flower petals. Place the fine-mesh screen on top of an old towel. Pour the pulpy mixture across the screen and spread it into an even, thin layer, blotting out any extra moisture. Let it dry overnight.

On the back of the card, share these instructions: "Soak the card overnight to activate the seeds; cut it into strips and plant them in a terra-cotta pot or in the ground, covering the strips with an inch (2.5 cm) of soil. Water the soil every day to keep it moist until the seeds start to sprout."

Makes 1 sheet of paper.

PARTY DECOR

Creating your own decorations with a variety of natural materials is a thoughtful and sustainable alternative to buying commercially produced decorations. Go DIY with materials like post-consumer paper products, repurposed fabrics, fresh flowers (preferably potted plants or dried flowers, see below), and other natural elements that are local and seasonal, like pine cones, branches, and shells. For larger events, consider renting decorations instead of buying new.

FLOWERS

Buy locally sourced, organic, and in-season flowers and have them wrapped in paper. If you can, grow your own buds in your garden or inside your home in terra-cotta or tin pots. To display cut flowers, place them in ceramic or glass mason jars, or a vase.

For big event and wedding centerpieces, use potted flowers and let guests take them home as party favors. As an alternative to fresh-cut flowers, try naturally dried and preserved flowers, which last much longer and can be more cost effective. Dried flowers also don't need to be refrigerated, so they give you one less thing to worry about on the day of the celebration.

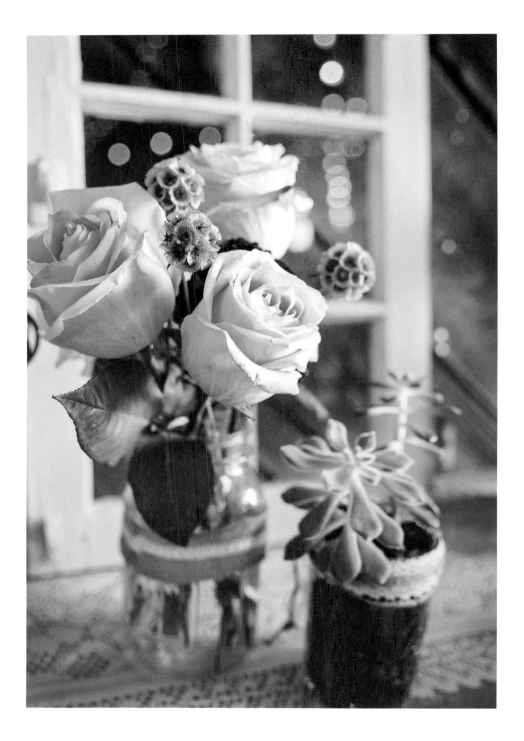

FESTIVE SIGNS

No biodegradable balloon option exists, which is why the promotional release of balloons has been banned in states such as California and Florida, and in places like Plymouth, England, and New South Wales, Australia. Planting a tree or flowers is a more eco-friendly and symbolic way to commemorate an event. You can also replace balloons with large cut-out letters or numbers, or with a hand-drawn sign.

Another option is to make your own bunting sign with colorful triangle flags. Repurpose fabric or buy scraps from a wholesale fabric supplier to make them, or use paper instead.

FACT Even a natural latex balloon still has chemicals, plasticizers, and dyes that are not biodegradable. Most airborne balloons or their bits and strings wind up in the ocean, where animals often mistake them for food or become entangled.

WHAT YOU'LL NEED

Multicolored fabric or paper scraps

11 feet (3.5 m) yarn or hemp rope

Needle and thread

On the fabric or paper, draw 15 same-size triangles with a base of 5 inches (13 cm) and a height of 8 inches (20 cm). Then cut them out with scissors and sew the base of each flag along the length of the yarn or hemp rope, leaving approximately 3½ inches (9 cm) of space between them. You can also add a handwritten letter to each flag to spell out a message. Hang the banner on the wall or above a doorway at your next fiesta!

TABLE LINENS

Choose tablecloths and napkins made from organic, natural, and durable fibers, preferably linen. You can make your own, too. Here's a simple method for making no-sew napkins; choose a colorful assortment of fabric or stick to a matching color scheme.

WHAT YOU'LL NEED

Fabric scraps (large enough for napkins) or about 2 yards
(2 m) linen

Preshrink the fabric by washing it in hot water and drying it. Cut it into 6 squares, about 12 × 12 inches (30 × 30 cm). Pull the threads out from all four edges to make a frayed fringe about ½ inch (1.5 cm) long. To keep the napkins from fraying further, line dry them after washing.

FACT Those quintessential red-checked picnic tablecloths at backyard barbecues and neighborhood pizza parlors are made from vinyl. PVC (RIC #3) plastic should be avoided at all costs as it's arguably the most toxic. Also avoid durable, high-absorbency paper napkins that don't tear easily, as they are made with nonwoven fabrics that contain plastic resins.

GIFTS

Instead of material goods, give your friends or family an experience or unique activity like a pottery class (where they can make a reusable mug), glow-in-the-dark bowling, an escape room, indoor rock climbing, or an improv class. Groupon, Eventbrite, and Airbnb offer good deals on experiential gifts. Inform the recipient of your gift via an email notice rather than a physical gift card made from PVC. If you don't know which type of experience the recipient would enjoy, consider donating to a charitable cause on his or her behalf.

FACT According to Finder, the top unwanted gifts are clothing and accessories (34 percent), household items (18 percent), and cosmetics and fragrances (14 percent). Plastic is ubiquitous in all of these categories.

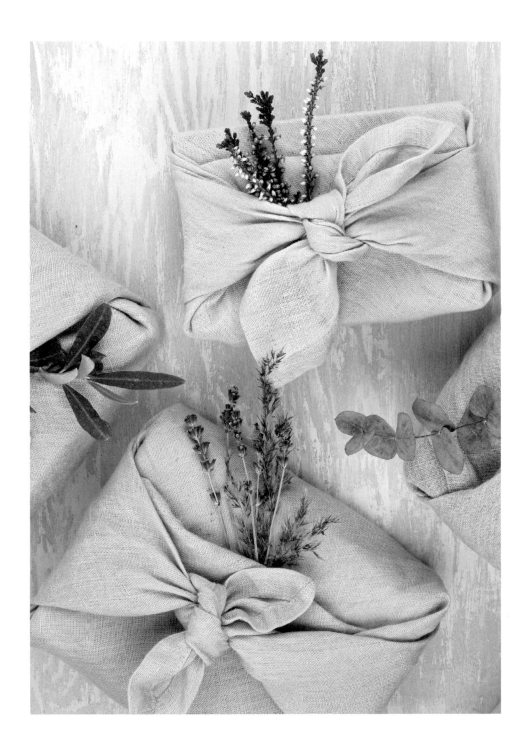

GIFT WRAP AND RIBBON

For holiday gifting, reuse last year's bags, gift wrap, and ribbons. If you must buy new, consider premade organic fabric gift bags that can be reused for decades. To close the bag, use jute twine and add branches, twigs, or dried flowers as decoration.

Another option is the traditional art of Japanese gift wrapping with cloth, known as *furoshiki*. It is elegant, easy, and environmentally friendly. Choose a square piece of lightweight but strong organic cloth three times longer at the diagonal than the gift. You can cut the square from an old bed sheet or use a bandanna or scarf (two gifts in one!). If you are using cut cloth, you can hem the edges for a cleaner look, or you can fray them (see page 196). Place the item you want to wrap on the cloth at a diagonal. Lift and lay the top and bottom corners over the gift. Then lift the remaining two corners and tie a double knot.

FACT Modern gift-wrapping paper can't be recycled because of its layered composition of paper with plastic in the form of glitter, gloss, and metallic coating. Ribbons are also a plastic-paper composite that can't be recycled and are disruptive at recycling centers, where they get caught in machines.

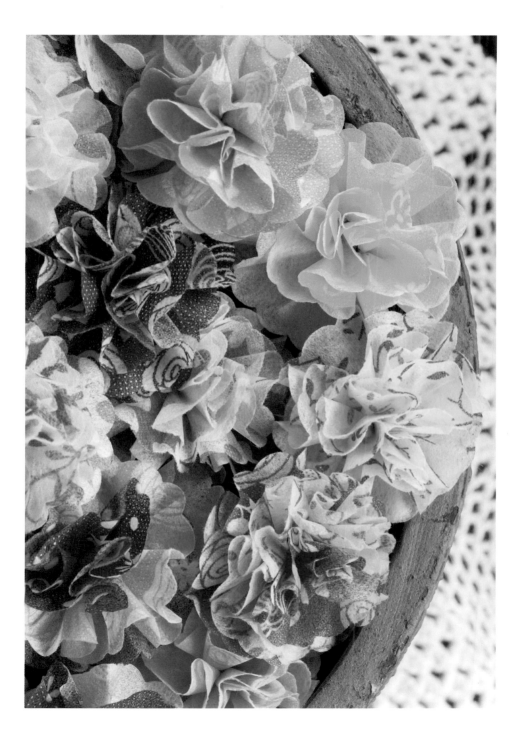

BIRTHDAY DECORATIONS

One of the most versatile and colorful materials for a birthday party is craft tissue paper. Use it to make decorative flowers or pom-poms or glue it on glass jars to make colorful luminaries. Choose a brand made from recycled paper pulp that is 100 percent biodegradable, which means it should have no sheen, glitter, or metallics. You can compost any scraps to avoid adding to the waste stream.

To make the pom-poms, simply use 4 sheets of tissue paper stacked on top of each other. Fold the stack in half and cut at the seam. Starting from one of the shorter edges, fold the entire length of the stack in an accordion fold in 1-inch (2.5 cm) increments. Trim the ends of the tissue into round or pointed tips. Then tie a string or wire securely in the center of this folded strip to create what looks like a bow-tie. Separate each layer, lifting the edges up and toward the middle, creating a blossoming flower.

PARTY FAVORS

A delicious way to thank your guests is with DIY treats instead of cheap, plastic trinkets. Bake batches of plain cookies or cupcakes to decorate with icing and sprinkles at the party (an activity and take-home gift all in one is a win-win for everyone!). Or, to avoid the sugar rush, set up a fun painting activity with natural eco-friendly paints (see Resources, page 236); the take-home gift is the painting.

GIFT BAGS

For a generous gift bag, give your guests reusable canvas bags and fill them with items such as bamboo toothbrushes, metal straws, a stainless-steel water bottle, chocolates wrapped in aluminum foil, and reusable cups (see Resources, page 242).

CELEBRATING FOR LUNAR NEW YEAR

To celebrate Lunar New Year, as they do in China and other parts of Asia, wear your finest and brightest clothes; red is the preferred color, symbolizing good fortune. It's also believed to ward off Nian, a lion-like horned beast who, according to legend, attacks villages every new year, eating crops, livestock, and even people, especially children. Don't have anything red? Shop at consignment stores for something that may not be brand-new (as the tradition goes) but is new to you. This is also an ideal time to declutter your own closet by donating items you no longer use to give them a second life.

FACT It's taboo to throw out the garbage on Lunar New Year Day, as it symbolizes tossing out good luck and fortune from the home.

VALENTINES

Cut back on plastic and paper waste by making edible Valentines such as heart-shaped conversation cookies (adorned with phrases like "Be Mine," "xoxo," or "Sweetheart"). A jar of homemade bath salts decorated with a handwritten label also makes a thoughtful, functional gift.

WHAT YOU'LL NEED

¾ cup (180 g) Epsom salt

¼ cup (65 g) pink Himalayan salt

¼ cup (45 g) baking soda

10 drops essential oil such as lavender

Dried flowers or herbs such as lavender, rose, calendula, sage, or mint (optional)

Place the salts, baking soda, and essential oils in a medium-size bowl and mix together with a wooden spoon. If you like, toss in a few heaping tablespoons of dried flowers or herbs for a colorful addition. Transfer the mixture to an airtight mason jar with a rubber seal. Store the jar in a cool, dark, and dry place, as bath salts absorb moisture easily when kept by the bathtub; stored this way, the salts will keep for 3 to 6 months.

Makes 1 cup (290 g).

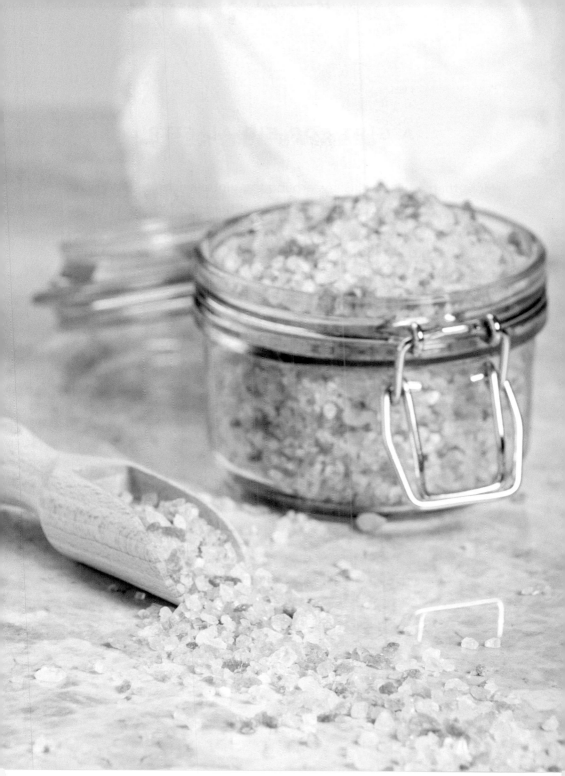

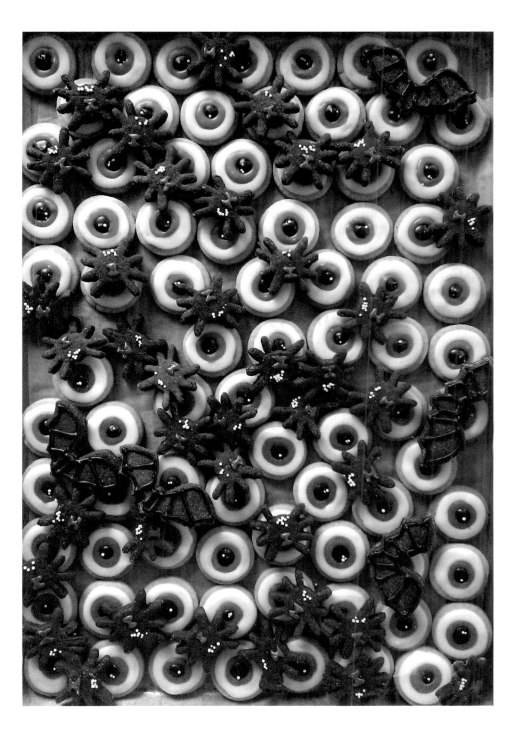

HALLOWEEN COSTUMES

Avoid the cheap, store-bought vinyl Halloween costume and be creative with items you already own. Raid your closet and dress as a pirate, rock star, *Men in Black* character, cheerleader, hippie, 1980s aerobics instructor, lumberjack, or other famous figure or fictional character.

TRICK OR TREATS

Treat trick-or-treaters to homemade cookies or the chocolates covered in foil that you find in the bulk bin section of your grocer. Foil is recyclable and a better option than individual plastic-wrapped candies, which are wasteful. Instead of using a plastic jack-o'-lantern, have your kids carry their treats in a pillowcase or homemade T-shirt bag (see page 20) decorated with spooky ghosts, bats, spiders, or goblins.

> **FACT** In the first half of the twentieth century, it was common for trick-or-treaters to receive coins, nuts, fruit, cookies, cakes, and toys. In the 1950s, candy producers started to market their products specifically as treats for Halloween, and by the 1970s individual-size candies wrapped in plastic became the main handout.

DIWALI LAMPS

The Hindu Festival of Lights highlights the triumph of good over evil and light over darkness. Use traditional earthenware oil lamps or make your own diyas using an orange peel to light up your home rather than plastic battery-operated lights.

WHAT YOU'LL NEED

1 orange

2 to 3 tablespoons olive oil or ghee

Use a knife to cut the orange around its circumference. Be careful not to cut too deep into the meat, keeping the bottom half of the skin and stem fully intact. Use your fingers to loosen the orange from the peel. Pour the oil into the empty half to about three-quarters full, and let it absorb fully into the stem wicks for about 5 minutes. Place on a plate and light the diya. As it is an open flame, keep an eye on it and keep it away from windy spots and flammable items. Extinguish the flame by blowing out the wick after 2 hours.

FACT A 23 percent increase of waste—an additional 5,291 tons in Delhi alone—in the form of plastic packaging from sweets, gifts, and firecrackers is generated before and during Diwali celebrations.

THANKSGIVING FEAST

The true meaning of Thanksgiving is giving thanks for the harvest. Celebrate by serving an array of fresh ingredients and seasonal veggies as opposed to frozen bags of vegetables and other processed foods. Head to the bulk bins for nuts, flour, and rice. If you have leftovers, offer guests mason jars and canvas totes to carry them home.

Homemade stuffing is easy to make and will taste so much better than anything you can find in a package.

WHAT YOU'LL NEED

1 loaf of bread, sliced

2 tablespoons olive oil

1 onion, peeled and diced

2 celery stalks, diced

¼ cup (4 g) parsley, chopped

1 teaspoon kosher salt

1 cup (120 g) chopped nuts (optional)

1 apple or pear, cored and diced (optional)

2 to 3 cups (475 to 720 ml) homemade stock or water

Cut the bread into 1-inch (2.5 cm) cubes and let it dry out overnight.

Preheat the oven to 350°F (175°C).

In a large frying pan, heat the oil over high heat and sauté the onion and celery for 5 minutes. Add the parsley, salt, and the day-old bread cubes, tossing to mix. If you want to make a fruit and nut stuffing, add the chopped nuts and apple or pear. Transfer the ingredients to a baking dish and pour in the water or stock. Cover with foil and bake for 45 minutes. Uncover and cook for an additional 20 minutes until golden brown on top.

Serves 10 to 12.

FACT The average American household generates 25 percent more waste per week between Thanksgiving and Christmas than the rest of the year, which translates into a million tons of extra garbage each week for a month.

HANUKKAH GELT

Light your menorah with package-free beeswax candles from the Package Free shop (see Resources, page 233) and buy dreidels made from natural wood (see Resources, page 242). For one of the eight nights, instead of giving an item as a gift, dedicate the night to charity by either donating money or planning a volunteer activity.

And skip the gelt (chocolate coins) packaged in plastic mesh bags and make your own Hanukkah-themed chocolates using a silicone mold.

2 4-ounce bars of dark chocolate chopped into small pieces, or 1 cup of chocolate chips from the bulk section of the supermarket

1 tablespoon of coconut oil or cocoa butter

Pinch of sea salt or 1 teaspoon chopped peanuts or other nuts, for flavoring

Silicone chocolate mold (see Resources, page 241)

Place the chocolate and coconut oil in a heatproof bowl suspended over a pan of simmering water. Make sure the bottom of the bowl is not touching the water. Stir the chocolate continuously for 2 to 3 minutes or until fully melted. Add a flavor element such as sea salt or nuts and continue to stir.

Fill each cavity of the mold with the melted chocolate up to the edge. Gently tap the tray a few times on your countertop to release air bubbles. Place the mold in the refrigerator and allow the chocolate to harden for at least 1 hour. Flip the mold over onto a clean surface and gently twist it to release the chocolates. If the coins aren't ready to come out, place the mold in the freezer for 5 minutes so the chocolate is extra firm. Package the coins in a jar or a holiday-themed tin. They will keep for 2 weeks in the refrigerator— if they last that long!

Makes 5 chocolates.

CHRISTMAS ORNAMENTS

Long before store-bought ornaments existed, Christmas trees were adorned with red apples, nuts, candles, and marzipan cookies. You can make natural decorations by stringing popcorn and cranberries and hanging foraged pinecones, red berry ilex branches, dried orange slices, or these ornaments made from flour dough.

FACT Artificial Christmas trees are made by slicing and fringing sheets of green PVC (RIC #3) plastic and attaching them to metal frames. The branches contain chemical adhesives and fire retardants. In California, some fake trees carry a required warning that the product contains certain hazardous chemicals known to cause cancer, birth defects, and other reproductive harm.

2 cups (280 g) all-purpose flour, plus additional for the work
*   surface*
1 cup (270 g) table salt
1 cup (240 ml) water
1 tablespoon oil
Natural Earth Paint (see page 236), optional

Preheat the oven to 300°F (150°C). Line a baking sheet with parchment paper.

In a large bowl, mix together the flour, salt, water, and oil. On a clean surface sprinkled with flour, roll the dough to ¼-inch (6 mm) thickness and use cookie cutters to form various shapes. Use a stainless-steel straw or a chopstick to make a small hole in the top of each ornament.

Place the cut-out shapes on the prepared pan and bake for 30 minutes. Let the ornaments cool completely before attaching a thread or a hook to the hole and hanging them on the tree. Or let them dry out for a few more days in open air before painting them.

This recipe will make 30 to 36 ornaments, depending on the size of the cookie cutter.

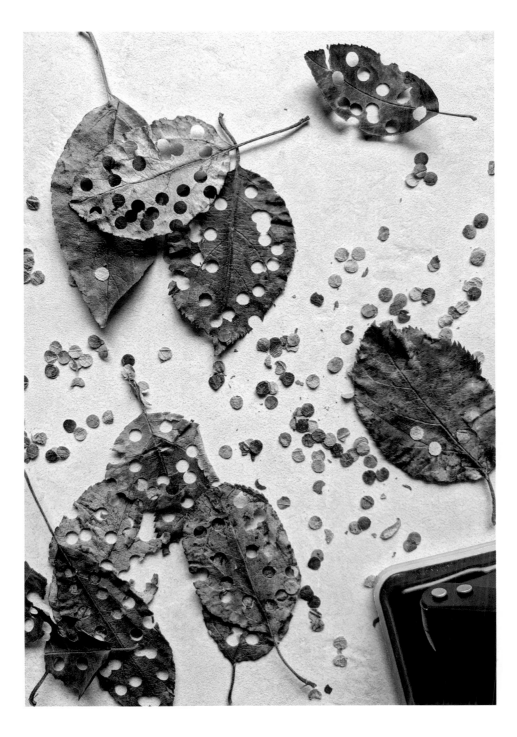

NEW YEAR'S EVE DECORATIONS

New Year's Eve, the most celebrated holiday around the world, is chock full of glitter to celebrate the possibilities of a bright new year. Mica, the original, natural glitter, is a shiny mineral that is mined from rock and ground into a sparkling powder that was found in Paleolithic cave paintings and Mayan temples. Modern-day glitter, made from etched aluminum bonded to polyethylene terephthalate, is a microplastic (less than ¼ inch/6 mm).

Always buy glitter made from non-GMO, biodegradable cellulose (see Resources, page 241). Or make your own biodegradable, compostable confetti using tissue paper or dried leaves and a hole-punch.

FACT Glitter is manufactured from sheets of Mylar, and when washed away, it enters water systems, moving past water treatment plants and into the ocean, where it winds its way up the food chain and onto our plates.

30-Day
Plastic Detox Plan

While there is undoubtedly plastic to be found in every part of daily life, the focus of this "detox" is on single-use plastic—items or packaging that is used only once and then tossed away. The idea is to refrain from buying anything new during this challenge, unless it's free from plastic packaging. Start the detox for yourself and then consider changes that you can implement for those in your care.

Studies have shown that it takes at least twenty-one days to form a new habit. This is applicable with integrating a plastic-free mind-set into your everyday life. Start any time, implement what you are able to, and add new baby steps each day. Being mindful doesn't mean feeling guilty each time you use plastic. As part of this exercise, you can also save all the plastic you go through each day for the month to see how much you accumulate.

Remember: Even if you refrain from using only one piece of new plastic each day, it's a step in the right direction.

WEEK ONE: **AT HOME**

Day 1. **Assess**

Start the detox by focusing on plastics at home and write down all the items that are made from "disposable" plastic. Include cling film and toiletries, and don't forget to look under the kitchen sink. Have kids or pets? Consider ways to minimize what plastics are currently incorporated in their lives. How many items are on your list?

Day 2. **Rethink**

When you run out of something, like food storage bags (see page 39) or laundry detergent (see page 54), challenge yourself by not restocking the same item. This forces you to rethink other package-free options for all items you use on a daily basis.

Day 3. **Reuse**

Look in your closets or cupboards for any reusable bags. Have them handy by your front door so you don't forget to grab a few before you leave your home. If you habitually put your fruits and vegetables into separate bags, consider purchasing a set of reusable cotton or mesh produce bags or make your own (see page 20).

Day 4. **Clean**

Keep your cleaning chemical-free and plastic-free by using a homemade solution of baking soda, vinegar, and water (see page 63) and store it in a glass container.

Day 5. **Fix**

Sew torn clothing, glue broken items, and fix any other objects that may be broken and only need a repair job. Borrow rather than buy something new. Moving forward, think twice about items you purchase. Is it something that you will keep for your lifetime or pass down to future generations?

Day 6. **Repurpose**

When you look around your home, what items do you keep but never use? If you haven't used the item in a year or two, most likely you will never use it, so release the clutter and repurpose these items by hosting a yard sale, going to a community swap, or donating them to a local charity.

Day 7. **Recycle**

Take a proactive stance with recycling at your home and workplace by becoming familiar with what plastics your local recycling center accepts and what are the best practices for preparing these items to be recycled. For example, do the containers need to be rinsed? Should you leave the caps on bottles? And is it necessary to remove stickers from the packaging first? Then debrief others at your home or office about what you learned.

WEEK TWO: **FOOD AND DRINK**

Day 8. **Hydrate naturally**

BYOBottle. Carry a stainless-steel or glass water bottle or jar with you and refill it throughout the day. Skip the sodas and juice boxes by adding fresh fruit to the water for a colorfully nutritious zing (see page 88).

Day 9. **Think outside the package**

Most packaged foods and drinks, even ones that aren't visibly in plastic, such as canned and frozen foods, milk cartons, ice-cream containers, and baby-food pouches, are made of several materials, including a layer of plastic to seal moisture in. Make these items from scratch at home (see pages 105, 94, 104, and 87) or buy them in reusable containers (see page 93).

Day 10. **Go nude**

At the supermarket, look for raw foods or fresh produce free from plastic packaging. Or better yet, discover what's available at farm- ers' markets, food co-ops, and international food shops, or partici- pate in community-supported agriculture (CSA).

Day 11. **Buy in bulk**

Bulk food stores are an old-but-new concept in which you can stock up on dry goods and pantry staples like legumes, grains, nuts, dried fruits, flour, sugar, cereal, snacks, and more. BYO container for this.

Day 12. **Dine in**

Cooking at home saves time and saves money and is better for your health. You can also make your own staples. Many of the most convenient foods are the simplest to make, like nut milks (see page 93), hummus, nut butters, tortillas, and more. Making them from scratch requires minimal ingredients, and they won't include any funky additives or shelf stabilizers . . . and it saves on using plastic packaging.

Day 13. **Refuse to use**

Refuse a plastic straw when you're at a restaurant or bar (see page 123) and bring your own container when you order takeout (see page 120). As more people become proactive, businesses will take note and try to be more accommodating, and maybe even offer incentives for bringing your own containers. If your favorite takeout places don't offer such a program, encourage them to start one.

Day 14. **Feed the earth**

Make less trash, especially food waste. Compost your food waste at home if you have the space (see page 65) or find out where you can drop off food scraps from your city's sanitation department (see Resources, page 235).

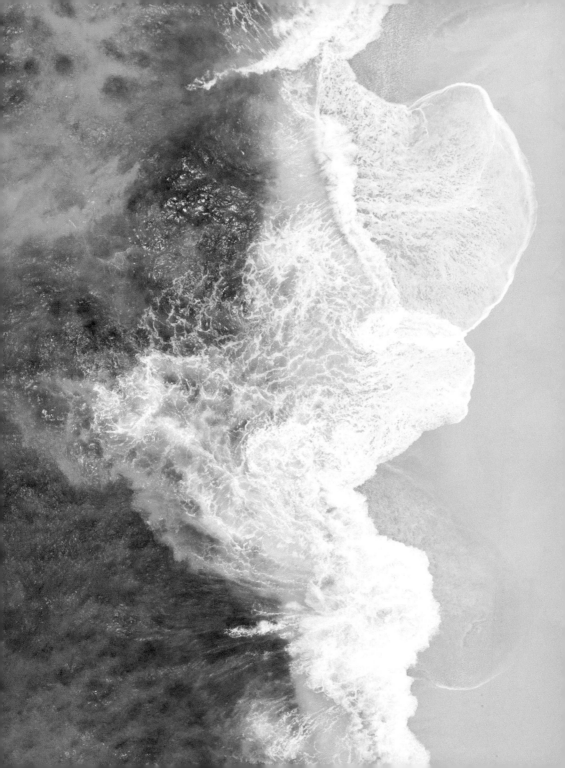

HALFWAY POINT CHECK-IN:

How are you doing with the detox plan? _____

_____

_____

_____

_____

What is most surprising? _____

_____

_____

_____

What is easiest? _____

_____

_____

_____

What is most challenging? _____

_____

_____

_____

Remember why your efforts are important. _____

_____

_____

_____

WEEK THREE: **HEALTH AND BEAUTY**

Day 15. **Raise the bar with personal care**

Choose to clean yourself with soap, shampoo, conditioner, and even body lotion in the form of a solid bar, or make your own at home (see pages 128–130).

Day 16. **Go minimal**

We actually don't need as many beauty products as marketing companies tell us we do. Determine which of your products are must-haves. By not having so many on hand, you will save time and also reduce the clutter in your bathroom.

Day 17. **Do-It-Yourself**

Making your own personal-care products can be as simple as brushing your teeth with plain old baking soda or moisturizing with coconut or almond oil.

Day 18. **Be beautiful from the inside out**

Hydrate your body by drinking plenty of water each day and by eating a diet full of fruits and vegetables. Health and beauty go beyond your skin and what products you use.

Day 19. **Choose quality over quantity**

While items like safety razors, menstrual cups, or period panties may initially seem expensive, the cost of these items are a fraction of how much "disposables" cost over a lifetime.

Day 20. **Don't flush!**

Stop flushing your contact lenses, tampons, and cotton swabs down the drain.

Day 21. **Be free (from chemicals)!**

By making your own deodorant (see page 141), toothpaste (see page 138), or moisturizers (see page 128), you are taking control and freeing yourself from many of the chemicals your body is exposed to on a daily basis.

WEEK 4: **ON THE GO**

Day 22. **Be prepared**

Plan ahead! If you are going to prepare a holiday feast, take plenty of bags to the market. Don't forget you will need enough bags for the bulk bin and produce section. Or if you're going to a food-tasting event, consider bringing a stainless-steel tumbler, utensils, and a reusable dish on which to receive samples.

Day 23. **Make it work**

Stash a coffee mug, a plate or a bowl (see page 178), and cutlery set (see page 121) in your desk at work. You should also keep a few reusable bags in a drawer in case you need them.

Day 24. **Stop and shop**

Shop at a brick-and-mortar store (a store in real life!) in order to avoid online packaging. If you must shop online, choose a company that can fulfill your request to have your shipment packaged with more sustainable options and without plastic or Styrofoam fillers.

Day 25. **Skip the receipt**

Go without receipts or go paperless by asking for an email receipt, or take a photo of the register screen for your records. If you do receive a paper receipt, don't recycle it.

Day 26. **Go natural!**

When shopping for clothing, either for work or working out, opt for sustainable materials like 100 percent organic cotton, hemp, or bamboo. Read the material label to avoid any synthetic fibers woven into fabrics (see page 30).

Day 27. **Skip the freebies**

Amusement parks, conventions, and food festivals can be overwhelming with the amount of waste they encourage. Enjoy the experience and don't buy into all the souvenirs, freebies, and takeaway samples.

Day 28. **Travel in style**

Make a checklist of reusable items to take when you travel. The list can include such things as headsets, bar shampoo, a reusable cup or bottle, bags, and a spork.

Day 29. **Make a statement**

Small actions that you take each day to avoid plastic might be so normal to you at this point that you won't think twice about it. You may find that refusing plastic and bringing your own reusables can create awareness and sometimes conversations. Share your experience and hopefully inspire others to do the same.

Day 30. **Celebrate (without the mess)!**

You did it! For a big way to give back, celebrate by organizing a community cleanup of a beach, river, lake, or other waterway or location. Plastic pollution can be found all over the globe, so you won't have to look far. Change can happen with just one person taking the initiative, and community will follow suit, actively aspiring to the same goal to make a positive change.

Congratulations on officially completing the 30-Day Detox! Now that you have created this positive mind-set, try to stick to those plastic-free habits. Don't be discouraged if you can't always avoid plastic. The important thing is to keep on doing what works for you and to share how your inspirational journey is helping the planet with friends, family, and colleagues.

RESOURCES

The following list of resources offers useful suggestions to purchase items that will help you reduce your plastic waste. When ordering online, ask retailers to ship their products to you without plastic packaging whenever possible.

GENERAL

EcoChoices Natural Living Store
   (ecochoices.com)
Environmental Working Group (ewg.org)
Loop (loopstore.com)
Life Without Plastic
   (lifewithoutplastic.com)
Package Free (packagefreeshop.com)
Preserve (preserve.eco)
TerraCycle Zero Waste Box
   (terracycle.com)
Unwrapped Life (unwrappedlife.com)
Wild Minimalist (wildminimalist.com)
The Zero Waste Collective
   (thezerowastecollective.com)

Water Bottles

Black + Blum (black-blum.com)
Hydro Flask (hydroflask.com)

Klean Kanteen (kleankanteen.com)
RefillMyBottle (refillmybottle.com)
Soma (drinksoma.com)
S'well (swell.com)
Takeya (takeyausa.com)
Tap (findtap.com)

Bags

Eco-Bags (ecobags.com)
Colony Co. (colonyco.com)
Credo Bags (credobags.com)
Khala & Co (khalaco.com)
Marley's Monsters
   (marleysmonsters.com)
Plastic bags and wraps recycling
   (plasticfilmrecycling.org)

AT HOME

Bed and Bath

Avocado Green Mattress
 (avocadogreenmattress.com)
Coyuchi (coyuchi.com)
EcoChoices Natural Living Store
 (ecochoices.com)
Eco Terra (ecoterrabeds.com)
Grund America (livegrund.com)
Happsy (happsy.com)
Jefferson Lane
 (jeffersonlanehome.com)
Natura (naturaworld.com)
Rawganique (rawganique.com)
Under the Canopy
 (underthecanopy.com)

Water Filters and Refill Stations

Black + Blum (blackblum.com)
Ippinka (ippinka.com)
Kishu Charcoal (kishucharcoal.com)
RefillMyBottle guide to refill stations
 (refillmybottle.com)
Tap app to find refill stations
 (findtap.com)

Clothing

Alexis Suitcase (alexissuitcase.com)
Black and Brown
 (shopblackandbrown.com)
Fyre Vintage (fyrevintage.com)
Poshmark (poshmark.com)
Rent the Runway (renttherunway.com)
The RealReal (therealreal.com)
ThredUP (thredup.com)
Tradesy (tradesy.com)

Kitchen

All-Clad (all-clad.com)
Anolon (anolon.com)
Bambu (bambuhome.com)
Bella (bellahousewares.com)
Bodum (bodum.com)
EcoJarz (ecojarz.com)
John Boos single-piece wooden cutting
 boards (johnboos.com)
Le Creuset (lecreuset.com)
Life Without Plastic
 (lifewithoutplastic.com)
Lodge Cast Iron (lodgemfg.com)
Oster Pro 1200 glass blender (oster.com)
Pyrex (pyrex.com)
Staub (zwilling.com/us/staub)

Baby Bottles

Evenflo Feeding (evenflofeeding.com)
Klean Kanteen (kleankanteen.com)
Lifefactory (lifefactory.com)
Philips Avent Natural (usa.philips.com)
Pura Kiki (purastainless.com/
 collections/baby)

Kids' Tableware and Cups

Bambu (bambuhome.com)
Coconut Bowls (coconutbowls.com)
EcoLunchbox (ecolunchboxes.com)
Munchkin (munchkin.com)

Baby Products

Lalabu bamboo bibs (lalabu.com)
Life Without Plastic
 (lifewithoutplastic.com)

Naturepedic crib mattresses
(naturepedic.com)
Our Green House (ourgreenhouse.com)
Soaring Heart organic crib mattress
(soaringheart.com)
Sprout furniture (sprout-kids.com)
TerraCycle Zero Waste Box
(terracycle.com)

Diapers

Amp Diapers (ampdiapers.com)
BabeeGreens (babeegreens.com)
BumGenius (bumgenius.com)
Charlie Banana (charliebanana.com)
Kawaii Baby (theluvyourbaby.com)

Pets

Arm & Hammer cat litter
(armandhammer.com/cat-litter)
Integrity (farmstore.com/product
-category/pet/cat-litter)
Ökocat cat litter (healthy-pet.com/
pages/okocat)
Package Free (packagefreeshop.com/
collections/pet-under-20)
Purrfectplay (purrfectplay.com)
Scoopeasy (scoopeasy.biz)
TerraCycle Zero Waste Box
(terracycle.com)
TLC Pet Food (tlcpetfood.com)

Cleaning Products and Supplies

Cleancult (cleancult.com)
Earth's Berries soap nuts
(earthsberries.com)
Guppyfriend (guppyfriend.com)
If You Care (ifyoucare.com)
Loop (loopstore.com)

Marley's Monsters
(marleysmonsters.com)
Mountain Rose Herbs aroma sprays,
herbal incense smudge sticks
(mountainroseherbs.com)
NaturOli soap nuts (naturoli.com)
Planet Wise reusable trash bag
(planetwiseinc.com)
Redecker (redecker.de)
Ten and Co. (tenandco.ca)
The Zero Waste Maker untowel kitchen
roll (the-zero-waste-maker.com)
Three Bluebirds (threebluebirds.com)
Waste Free Products laundry paste and
soap (wastefreeproducts.com)
Who Gives a Crap
(us.whogivesacrap.org)
Wild Minimalist (wildminimalist.com/
collections/cleaning)

Composting and Gardening

Eartheasy (learn.eartheasy.com/guides/
composting)
FoodCycler (nofoodwaste.com)
Guide to composting—USA (litterless
.com/wheretocompost)
Jora Composters (joracomposters.com)
Plantz4U2 (etsy.com/shop/Plantz4U2)
Western Pulp floral and nursery
containers (westernpulp.com)

Home Entertainment and Electronics

CD Recycling Center of America
(cdrecyclingcenter.org)
Earth 911 recycling (earth911.com)
Electronics TakeBack Coalition
(electronicstakeback.com)

GreenDisk (greendisk.com)

Second Spin (secondspin.com)

TerraCycle Zero Waste Box
(terracycle.com)

Toys and Games

Bears for Humanity
(bearsforhumanity.com)

Begin Again (beginagaintoys.com)

Big Future Toys (bigfuturetoys.com)

Elly Lu (ellylu.com)

Oli & Carol (oliandcarol.com/us)

PlanToys (usa.plantoys.com)

Taraluna (taraluna.com)

Under the Nile (underthenile.com/
collections/toys)

Arts and Crafts

Natural Earth Paint
(naturalearthpaint.com)

Old Fashioned Milk Paint Co.
(milkpaint.com)

Stockmar Beeswax Crayons
(bellalunatoys.com)

Packing Materials

EcoEnclose (ecoenclose.com)

Ecovative Design mushroom packaging
(ecovativedesign.com)

Life Without Plastic potato starch glue
paste (lifewithoutplastic.com)

Ranpak Geami WrapPak (ranpak.com)

Uline cushion wrap roll (uline.com)

Western Pulp Products
(westernpulp.com)

Refillable Fountain Pens and Mechanical Pencils

Diplomat (diplomat-pen.com)

Faber-Castell (faber-castell.com)

Kaweco (kaweco-pen.com/en)

Parker (parkerpen.com/en-US/
fountain-pen)

Waterman (waterman.com)

Printer Cartridges

Earth911 recycling (earth911.com)

TerraCycle Zero Waste Box
(terracycle.com)

FOOD AND DRINK

Food

CSAs, farmers' markets and food
co-ops—USA (localharvest.org)

Imperfect Foods (imperfectfoods.com)

Pick-your-own farms—USA
(pickyourown.org)

Zero-waste grocery guide—global
(bepakt.com)

Zero-waste grocery guide—USA
(litterless.com/wheretoshop)

Drinks

Adagio Teas porcelain mug and infuser
(adagio.com)

Drink Milk in Glass Bottles
milk delivery—USA
(drinkmilkinglassbottles.com)

Dwell Tea Co (cwellteaco.com)

Ekobrew reusable K-Cup (ekobrew.com)

English Tea Store tea strainers (englishteastore.com)

Keep Cup (keepcup.com)

M*lkman nut milk delivery—England (mlkman.com)

NotMilk NYC delivery (notmilknyc.com)

SodaStream (sodastream.com)

Soma brew cup and ceramic mug (drinksoma.com)

Steelys stainless-steel growler (steelysdrinkware.com)

Toast Ale (toastale.com)

WayCap reusable coffee pods (compatible-capsules.com)

Wild Minimalist nut milk bags and reusable coffee filters (wildminimalist.com)

Yogurt

GT'S CocoYo coconut yogurt (gtslivingfoods.com/offering/cocoyo/pure-2/)

Nounós Creamery Greek yogurt (nounoscreamery.com)

Oui by Yoplait French-style yogurt (ouibyyoplait.com)

St. Benoit Creamery pasture-raised milk yogurt (stbenoit.com)

Frozen Food

Field Fare—UK (field-fare.com)

Teva Deli vegan burgers (loopstore.com/brand/teva-deli)

Onyx Containers ice cube trays and ice pop molds (onyxcontainers.com)

Pasta and Noodles

Puretto spaghetti, whole wheat penne, and angel hair pasta (loopstore.com; some bulk dry-goods bins will sell loose pasta, soba, and udon by weight)

Gum

Chicza (chiczausa.com)

Glee Gum (gleegum.com)

Simply Gum (simplygum.com)

True Gum (truegum.com)

Lunches and Snacks

Abeego (abeego.com)

Black + Blum (black-blum.com)

Colony Co (colonyco.com)

ECOlunchbox (ecolunchboxes.com)

If You Care unbleached bags (ifyoucare.com)

LunchBots (lunchbots.com)

LunchSkins reusable zippered bags (lunchskins.com)

PlanetBox (planetbox.com)

Stasher silicone storage bags (stasherbag.com)

Steelys Drinkware steel containers and lunchboxes (steelysdrinkware.com)

U-Konserve (ukonserve.com)

Utensils

Bambu (bambuhome.com)

Life Without Plastic (lifewithoutplastic.com)

Package Free (packagefreeshop.com)

To-Go Ware (to-goware.com)

Straws

Hay! Straws (haystraws.com)
Loliware (loliware.com)
SeaStraws (seastraws.co)
Simply Straws (simplystraws.com)
Steelys Drinkware
  (steelysdrinkware.com)
S'wheat (swheatstraws.com)

Disposable Plates

Bambu (bambuhome.com)
Made by Leaf (madebyleaf.com)

Freezer Packs

Plastic Free stainless-steel ice pack
  (packagefreeshop.com)
The Tickle Trunk steel ice cubes and
  packs (thetickletrunk.com)

Coolers

Go Plastic Free vintage-style cooler
  (https://plasticfree.store)
Igloo Recool (igloocoolers.com/pages/
  recool)

HEALTH AND BEAUTY

Environmental Working Group (ewg.org)
Preserve (www.preserve.eco)
TerraCycle (terracycle.com)
Wild Minimalist (wildminimalist.com/
  collections/health-beauty)

Moisturizers

Bee Love Buzz (beelovebuzz.com)
Booda Organics (boodaorganics.com)
Flora almond oil (florahealth.com)
Garden of Life coconut oil
  (gardenoflife.com)
Meow Meow Tweet
  (meowmeowtweet.com)
Organic Essence (organic-essence.com)
Viva Naturals shea butter
  (vivanaturals.com)

Soaps

Ethique (ethique.com)
Linear Beauty (linearbeauty.com)
Lush (lush.com)
Meow Meow Tweet
  (meowmeowtweet.com)
Shea Moisture African black soap
  (sheamoisture.com)
Soaptopia (soaptopia.com)

Shampoos and Conditioners

Badger shampoo bar (badgerbalm.com)
Chagrin Valley Soap and Salve Company
  (chagrinvalleysoapandsalve.com)
Ethique (ethique.com)
Plaine Products (plaineproducts.com)

Combs, Hairbrushes, and Hair Ties

Kooshoo organic cotton hair ties
  (kooshoo.com)
Life Without Plastic brush and comb
  (lifewithoutplastic.com)
Package Free (packagefreeshop.com)
PureGLO (pureglonaturals.com)

Hair Products

Badger hair pomade
    (badgerbalm.com)
Captain Blankenship Mermaid Sea
    Salt Hair Spray (captainblankenship
    .com)
Jim + Henry Buy Five (jimandhenry.
    com/buy/five-250ml-pre-order)
Lush henna hair dyes (lush.com)
Mountain Rose Herbs henna and herbal
    hair color (mountainroseherbs.com)

Oral Care

Bite (bitetoothpastebits.com)
Brush with Bamboo toothbrush
    (brushwithbamboo.com)
Davids Premium Natural Toothpaste
    (davids-usa.com)
Dental Lace refillable dental floss
    (dentallace.com)
Georganics mouthwash tablets
    and oil pulling mouthwash
    (georganics.com)
Lucky Teeth (lucky-teeth.com)
Simplifeied (simplifeied.com)

Deodorants

Blk + Grn (blkgrn.com)
Lush deodorant bars and dusting
    powders (lush.com)
Meow Meow Tweet deodorant sticks
    and creams (meowmeowtweet.com)
Pretty Frank (pretty-frank.com)

Shaving and Grooming

Albatross Designs razors
    (albatrossdesigns.it)

Booda Butter shaving cream
    (boodaorganics.com)
MOOM (thenaturalshop.co.uk/moom
    -classic-hair-remover-kit-refill-with
    -tea-tree-oil)
Oui The People (ouithepeople.com)
Parissa (parissa.com)
Rockwell Razors (getrockwell.com)
Wet Shaving Products
    (wetshavingproducts.com)

Cosmetics

Axiology (axiologybeauty.com)
Elate Cosmetics (elatebeauty.com)
Kjaer Weis (kjaerweis.com)
Origins (origins.com)

Cotton Squares

Marley's Monsters
    (marleysmonsters.com)
Öko Créations makeup removal pads
    (okocreations.ca)
The Zero Waste Maker (the-zero-waste
    -maker.com)

Cotton Swabs/Curettes

Humankind (byhumankind.com)
Hydrophil (hydrophil.com/en)
LastSwab (lastobject.com)
The Humble Co. (thehumble.co/
    cotton-swabs)
YesCool Ear Curette (etsy.com/shop/
    YesCool)

Toilet Paper

Plastic Film Recycling
    (plasticfilmrecycling.org)
Reel (reelpaper.com)

Seventh Generation
(seventhgeneration.com)
Who Gives a Crap (whogivesacrap.org)

Handkerchiefs

HankyBook (hankybook.com)
Life Without Plastic
(lifewithoutplastic.com)
The Zero Waste Maker (the-zero-waste
-maker.com)

Feminine Care

DivaCup (divacup.com)
Lunette Menstrual Cups
(lunette.com)
OrganiCup (organicup.com)
Period Aisle (periodaisle.com)
The Moon Cup (mooncup.com)
Thinx period-proof underwear
(shethinx.com)

Sunscreens

All Good sunscreen butter
(allgoodproducts.com)

Eir Surf Mud (eirnyc.com)
Meow Meow Tweet
(meowmeowtweet.com)
Raw Elements (rawelementsusa.com)

Insect Repellents

Badger (badgerbalm.com)
Meow Meow Tweet
(meowmeowtweet.com)

Bandages

Patch (us.patchstrips.com)

Earplugs

Ohropax (ohropax.de/en)

Contact Lenses and Contact Lens Solution

Bausch + Lomb One by One Recycling
Program (biotrueonedaylenses.com/
one-by-one-recycling)
TerraCycle (terracycle.com/en-US/
brigades/bauschrecycles)

ON THE GO

Receipts and Tickets

Apple Pay (apple.com/apple-pay)
Atom Tickets (atomtickets.com)
Expensify (expensify.com)
Fandango (fandango.com)
Google Pay (pay.google.com)
PayPal (paypal.com)
Ticketmaster (ticketmaster.com)
Venmo (venmo.com)

Phone Case

Carved (carved.com)
Pela Case (pelacase.com)

Travel

Earthworks System to return PVC hotel
key cards (earthworkssystem.com/
consumers.html)

Green Hotels Association
(greenhotels.com)
Green Travel roundup (usgbc.org/
articles/green-travel-roundup
-leedcertified-places-see)
LEED-certified hotels (readymag.com/
usgbc/hospitality/where)
Life Without Plastic metal travel jar kit
(lifewithoutplastic.com)
Marley headphones
(thehouseofmarley.com)
Package Free zero waste travel kit
(packagefreeshop.com)
Samsonite eco suitcases
(shop.samsonite.com)
Steelys Drinkware steel flasks
(steelysdrinkware.com)

Hand Sanitizer
Weller Tribe (wellertribe.com)

Footwear
Ecoalf sneakers and flip-flops
(ecoalf.com)
Feelgoodz rubber flip-flops
(feelgoodz.com)
Native shoes, boots, and sandals
(nativeshoes.com)
Soles 4 Souls donations
(soles4souls.org)
Sustain Your Style
(sustainyourstyle.org)
Veja sneakers (veja-store.com)

Lighters
Tesla Coil Lighters
(teslacoillighters.com)
Zippo (zippo.com)

Yoga Mat
42 Birds (42birds.com)
Jade Yoga (jadeyoga.com)
Manduka (manduka.com)

SPECIAL OCCASIONS

TerraCycle Party Decorations Zero
Waste Box (terracycle.com)

Party Invitations and Greeting Cards
Aya Paper (ayapaper.co)
Botanical Paper Works
(botanicalpaperworks.com)
Earth Hero seeding cards (earthhero
.com/brands/seeding-cards)
Evite (evite.com)

Natural Earth Paint
(naturalearthpaint.com)
Paperless Post (paperlesspost.com)

Decorations
BioGlitz (bioglitz.co)
Botanical Paper Works biodegradable
confetti (botanicalpaperworks.com)
Glitra glitter (glitra.org)
Glitterevolution
(glitterevolution.com)

Green Packaging Group recycled tissue
paper (greenpackaginggroup.com/
paper)

GFTWoodcraft (etsy.com/shop/
GFTWoodcraft)

Hanukkah-theme silicone mold
(lavendersbakeshop.com/products/
hanukkah-theme)

RusticWoodSlices (etsy.com/shop/
rusticwoodslices)

Snuggly Monkey wooden Easter eggs
(snugglymonkey.com)

StoneHouseCrafts (etsy.com/shop/
stonehousecrafts)

Wooden dreicels (etsy.com/market/
wood_dreidel)

Table Linens

Fog Linen Work (shop-foglinen.com)

LinenLifeIdeas (etsy.com/shop/
linenlifeideas)

Package Free organic cloth napkins
(packagefreeshop.com)

Gifts

Groupon (groupon.com)

LivingSocial (livingsocial.com)

Package Free bath salts
(packagefreeshop.com)

Gift Wrap and Gift Bags

Cotton & Canvas Company wine and
favor bags (cottonandcanvasco
.com)

TheFabWrap (etsy.com/shop/
thefabwrap)

Gladfolk (wearegladfolk.com)

VadelmaCreations furoshiki (etsy.com/
shop/vadelmacreations)

SOURCES

INTRODUCTION

Combs and Billiard Balls
smithsonianmag.com/smart-news/once
-upon-time-exploding-billiard-balls
-were-everyday-thing-180962751/

Ford Soybean Car
autonews.com/cars-concepts-history/
ford-introduces-first-plastic-soybean
-car

Leo Baekeland
sciencehistory.org/historical-profile/
leo-hencrik-baekeland

Volume of Plastic Over the Years
Edward Humes, *Garbology: Our Dirty
Love Affair with Trash* (New York:
Avery, 2012)
nationalgeographic.com/magazine
/2018/06/plastic-planet-waste-
pollution-trash-crisis/

Plastic in the Ocean
ellenmacarthurfoundation.org/assets/
downloads/EllenMacArthurFoundation
_NewPlasticsEconomy_21-1-2016.pdf

Recycling
unenvironment.org/interactive/beat-
plastic-pollution/

Water Bottles
utahrecycles.org/get-the-facts/the-facts-
plastic/

Bags
theworldcounts.com/counters/waste_
pollution_facts/plastic_bags_used_
per_year

Petrochemical Plants and Health Issues
www.washingtonpost.com/archive/
politics/1987/12/22/jobs-and-illness
-in-petrochemical-corridor/e623deeb
-c966-47fe-867d-b395046726d1/

Mattresses
motherjones.com/politics/2008/03/
  should-you-ditch-your-chemical-
  mattress/

Shower Curtains
Beth Terry, *Plastic-Free* (New York:
  Skyhorse Publishing, 2012)

Bed and Bath Linens
businessinsider.com/how-tencel
  -compares-to-cotton-2015-9

Clothing
greenpeace.org/archive-international/
  Global/international/briefings/toxics
  /2016/Fact-Sheet-Timeout-for-fast
  -fashion.pdf

Kitchen Cookware
foodmatters.com/article/is-your-cook
  ware-safe

Cutting Boards
nestandglow.com/life/wood-chopping
  -board-better-plastic

Water Filters
bottledwater.org/public/BMC2017_
  BWR_StatsArticle.pdf

Napkins and Towels
theatlantic.com/family/archive/2018/12/
  paper-towels-us-use-consume/577672/

Wax Food Wraps
Edward Humes, *Garbology: Our Dirty
  Love Affair with Trash* (New York:
  Avery, 2012)

learn.eartheasy.come/articles/is-food-
  packaging-safe/

Baby Wipes
onegreenplanet.org/news/wet-wipes-
  made-plastic-uk-wants-banned/

Diapers
phys.org/news/2019-02-vanuatu-
  disposable-diapers-flush.html

Dry Cleaning
huffingtonpost.com/stefanie-michaels/
  eco-friendly-cleaning-bag_b_160730.
  html

Trash Bags
transparencymarketresearch.com/
  garbage-bag-market.html

Air Fresheners
content.time.com/time/health/
  article/0,8599,1664954,00.html

Cleaning Products
ec.europa.eu/environment/chemicals/
  reach/pdf/39168%20Intentionally%20
  added %20microplastics%20-%20
  Final%20report%2020171020.pdf

Electronics
who.int/ceh/risks/ewaste/en/
sciencedirect.com/science/article/pii/
  S2452223618300452

Toys and Games
huffingtonpost.com/entry/your-kids-
  toys-are-killing-the-planet_us
  _58ffa383e4b0f5463a1a9472

eluxemagazine.com/magazine/playing
-with-fire-the-hidden-dangers-of-
toys/

Packing Materials

latimesblogs.latimes.com/greenspace
/2011/06/foam-takeout-containers-
ban-styrofoam-california.html
theatlantic.com/business/
archive/2016/12/air-cushions/511487/

Printer Cartridge

agreenerrefill.com/FAQs

Pens

u osu.edu/bicpens/05-consumption/

Tape

scotchbrand.com/3M/en_US/scotch-
brand/products/all-tape/

Gardening Pots

mobot.org/hort/activ/plasticpots.shtml
gardenersworld.com/how-to/gardening-
with-less-plastic/

TWO   **FOOD AND DRINK**

Introduction

nationalgeographic.com/magazine/
2018/06/plastic-planet-waste-
pollution-trash-crisis/

Baby Food and Drinks

psmag.com/environment/consumers
-love-squeezable-plastic-pouches-for
-foodtoo-bad-recyclers-hate-them
nrdc.org/experts/peter-lehner/fast
-food-trash-nation-time-cut-down
-packaging-waste

Drinks

https://www.theatlantic.com/national
/archive/2013/03/americans-drink-44
-gallons-soda-year/317523/
slate.com/articles/health_and_science
/map_of_the_week/2012/07/map_of
_soda_consumpt on_americans_drink
_more_than_anyone_else.html

Coffee

http://action.storyofstuff.org/sign/
amount-k-cups-have-been-thrown
-landfills-could-wrap-around-planet
-over-11-times

Tea

theatlantic.com/health/archive/2013/04
/are-tea-bags-turning-us-into-plastic
/274482/

Meat and Seafood

cancer.org/cancer/cancer-causes/
general-info/known-and-probable-
human-carcinogens.html

Bread

ewg.org/research/nearly-500-ways
-make-yoga-mat-sandwich
history.com/news/a-brief-history-of-
bread

Yogurt

prnewswire.com/news-releases/us
   -yogurt-market-sales-approach-9
   -billion-at-retail-growth-expected
   -through-2022-says-packaged-facts
   -report-380581615.html

Condiments

tedium.co/2016/01/07/condiment-sauce
   -packet-squeeze/

Gum

www.npr.org/templates/story/story.
   php?storyId=106439600

Takeout Containers

plasticpollutioncoalition.org/guides-eats/

Utensils

wholefoodsmagazine.com/blog/ending
   -take-out-waste/

Straws

nytimes.com/2018/07/19/business/plastic
   -straws-ban-fact-check-nyt.html

THREE   **HEALTH AND BEAUTY**

Introduction

abcnews.go.com/Health/women-put
   -average-168-chemicals-bodies-day
   -consumer/story?id=30615324
chemicalsinourlife.echa.europa.eu/
   chemicals-in-cosmetics
makeup-in.com/05-trends-en/korean
   -women-use-more-than-thirteen
   -beauty-products-per-day/
blog.beautycounter.com/why-
   beautycounter-bans-more-ingredients
   -than-the-u-s/

Shampoos and Conditioners

simplemost.com/solid-shampoo
   -eliminates-plastic-packaging/
statista.com/statistics/254608/global
   -hair-care-market-size/
unwrappedlife.com/blogs/blog/end
   -plastic-pollution-for-earth-day

Combs and Hair Brushes

atlasobscura.com/articles/unbreakable
   -comb-history
nationalgeographic.com/magazine
   /2018/06/plastic-planet-waste-
   pollution-trash-crisis/

Hair Gel and Spray

aol.it/2yi0yuP

Hair Color

chemicalsinourlife.echa.europa.eu/good
   -to-know-about-hair-dyes
sierraclub.org/sierra/what-
   environmental-impact-hair-dye

Toothbrushes

nationalgeographic.com/environment
   /2019/06/story-of-plastic-toothbrushes/

Toothpaste

1millionwomen.com.au/blog/why-i-quit
-toothpaste/
blog.stpub.com/bid/204975/Brushing
-Off-Wasteful-Packaging

Deodorants

smithsonianmag.com/history/how
-advertisers-convinced-americans
-they-smelled-bad-12552404/

Razors

greenmatters.com/living/2017/09/25/
Z1oInGt/razors-ocean

Cosmetics

independent.co.uk/news/long_reads
/beauty-industry-plastic-pollution
-environment-climate-change
-cosmetics-a8697951.html

Handkerchiefs

envisioningtheamericandream.com
/2014/02/27/colds-flu-and-the-story
-of-kleenex/
greengroundswell.com/paper-facial
-tissue-history-and-environmental
-impact/2013/12/05/

Feminine Care

thedailybeast.com/save-the-planet-
ditch-the-tampon
groundswell.org/women-spend-hundreds
-of-extra-dollars-per-year-heres-one
-easy-out/

Sunscreens

nationalgeographic.com/travel/features/
sunscreen-destroying-coral-reefs
-alternatives-travel-spd/

Contact Lenses

bbc.com/news/science-environment
-45222865

FOUR ON THE GO

Susan Freinkel, *Plastic: A Toxic Love
Story* (New York: Houghton Mifflin
Harcourt, 2011)
nationalgeographic.com/magazine
/2018/06/plastic-planet-waste-
pollution-trash-crisis

Receipts and Tickets

scientificamerican.com/article/just-how
-harmful-are-bisphenol-a-plastics/

Business Cards

creditconkey.com/business-card
-statistics.html
japantimes.co.jp/life/2017/05/06
/lifestyle/calling-card-evolution
-business-cards-japan/#.XIsdSqhKg2w

Travel Headsets

apex.aero/2019/02/21/sound-tube-
history-airline-headsets

Travel Toiletries

greenhotelier.org/our-themes/waste
  -management/

Hotel Key Cards

cdn2.hubspot.net/hubfs/455144/Investor
  %20Pages/Resources/OpenKey%20
  Infographic%20V1.8.pdf

Coolers

miami.cbslocal.com/2017/06/13/miami
  -dade-styrofoam-ban-starts-july-1/

Athletic Shoes

weforum.org/agenda/2018/04/these
  -eco-friendly-sneakers-are-made-from
  -plants/

FIVE SPECIAL OCCASIONS

Festive Signs

Capt. Charles Moore, *Plastic Ocean* (New
  York: Penguin Group, 2011)
balloonsblow.org/laws-concerning
  -balloons/

Gifts

finder.com/unwanted-gifts

Trick or Treats

theatlantic.com/health/archive/2010/10
  /how-candy-and-halloween-became
  -best-friends/64895/

Diwali Lamps

timesofindia.indiatimes.com/city/indore
  /your-diwali-discards-raise-citys
  -waste-output-by-23/articleshow
  /71748004.cms
newslaundry.com/2016/11/12/how-delhis
  -air-pollution-was-made-worse-by-
  diwali-trash

Thanksgiving Feast

lbre.stanford.edu/pssistanford-recycling
  /frequently-asked-questions/frequently
  -asked-questions-holiday-waste
  -prevention

ACKNOWLEDGMENTS

It was the award-winning documentary *A Plastic Ocean* that inspired and led us both to a plastic-free journey and this amazing collaboration. *Living Without Plastic* would not have been possible without the support and encouragement of Leigh Eisenman, who envisioned the need for a practical handbook to promote awareness about how to reduce single-use plastic. We want to also thank Judy Pray and Artisan Books for their belief in the need for creating this beautiful book. Most importantly, we thank you, reader, for embarking on this journey with us and inspiring positive change.

PHOTO CREDITS

Christine Wong: Page 2 (title page), page 18 (Water Bottles), page 21 (Bags), page 34 (Kitchen Utensils), page 61 (Sponges), page 62 (Cleaning Products), page 71 (Arts and Crafts), page 72 (Packing Materials), page 86 (Baby Food and Drinks), page 92 (Nut and Seed Milks), page 97 (Fruit), page 106 (Pasta and Noodles), page 111 (Breakfast Cereal), page 114 (Trail Mix and Snack Bars), page 119 (School Lunches and Snacks), page 122 (Straws), page 129 (Moisturizers), page 143 (Razors), page 147 (Cotton Squares), page 152 (Sunscreens), page 180 (Meals and Snacks On the Go), page 185 (Yoga Mats), page 208 (Halloween Costumes), page 211 (Diwali Lamps), page 218 (New Year's Eve Decorations)

Stock Photography: Page 22-23 (At Home): Photographee.eu/Shutterstock.com; page 28 (Bed and Bath Linen): World_of_Textiles/Shutterstock.com; page 33 (Kitchen Cookware): Iryna Melnyk/Shutterstock.com; page 40 (Wax Food Wraps): NiniPanini/Shutterstock.com; page 44 (Kids' Tableware and Cups): New Africa/Shutterstock.com; page 49 (Diapers): Auribe/Shutterstock.com; page 50 (Pet Food): Sharaf Maksumov/Shutterstock.com; page 55 (Laundry): Aneta_Gu/Shutterstock.com; page 58 (Air Fresheners): amyjohnsonphoto/Adobe Stock; page 64 (Composting): Daisy Daisy/Shutterstock.com; page 68 (Toys and Games): Rawpixel.com/Shutterstock.com; page 77 (Pens): besjunior/Adobe Stock; page 80 (Gardening Pots): Bogdan Sonjachnyj/Shutterstock.com; page 82-83 (Food and Drink): Photographee.eu/Shutterstock.com; page 89 (Drinks): Antonina Vlasova/Shutterstock.com; page 101 (Bread): Pia Violeta Pasat/Shutterstock.com; page 124-125 (Health and Beauty): Natalia Klenova/Shutterstock.com; page 136 (Toothbrushes): Lazy_Bear/Shutterstock.com; page 154 (Insect Repellents): Angelina Zinovieva/Shutterstock.com; page 160-161 (On the Go): TierneyMJ/Shutterstock.com; page 168 (Travel): cktravelling/Shutterstock.com; page 173 (Hotel Mini Bar): Thiraphon 3839/Shutterstock.com; page 177 (Coolers): Roschetzky Photography/Shutterstock.com; page 186-187 (Special Occasions): bearmoney /Adobe Stock; page 193 (Party Decor): Angela/Adobe Stock; page 198 (Gift Wrap and Ribbon): Netrun78/Shutterstock.com; page 200 (Birthday Decorations): Sagun Tongnim/Shutterstock.com; page 205 (Valentines): EasterBunny/Shutterstock.com; page 226 (Halfway Point Check-In): Pongtap/Adobe Stock

INDEX

A

accessories, pet, 53
air fresheners, 59
appliances, kitchen, 31
arts and crafts, 70–71,
   236
athletic shoes, 182, 241

B

baby products
  about: overview of non-
    plastic alternatives, 46;
    resources, 234–235
  bottles, 43, 234
  diapers, 48–49
  food and drinks, 87
  wipes, 47
Baekeland, Leo, 10
bags, grocery/produce,
   etc., 20, 233
Bakelite, 10
bandages, 156, 240
baskets, Easter, 207
bed and bath. See also
   cleaning solutions
   and supplies; clothing;
   health and beauty
  about: resources, 234
  air fresheners, 59
  linens, 29
  mattresses, 26

  shower curtains, 27
  toilet paper, 149, 239
beer, 95
bioplastics, 13, 57
birthdays. See special
   occasions
bottles
  baby, 43, 234
  drinks, 88
  water, 19, 233
BPA (Bisphenol A), 31, 38,
   42, 51, 53, 164
BPS (Bisphenol S), 38,
   45, 51
bread, 100–101
breakfast cereal, 110–111
business cards, 165

C

cats. See pets
cellulose, plastic from, 9–10
cereal, 110–111
cheese, 108
chewing gum, 117
Christmas ornaments,
   216–217
cleaning solutions and
   supplies. See also
   health and beauty
  about: natural cleaning
   products, 63

  laundry, 29, 30, 54–55
  resources, 235
  sponges, 60–61
clothing
  about: resources, 234
  athletic shoes, 182, 241
  buying new, 30
  dry cleaning, 56
  laundry, 29, 30, 54–55
coffee, 90
coloring hair, 135
combs and hairbrushes,
   132, 238
composting, 65, 236
condiments, 109
conditioners, shampoos
   and, 131, 238
contact lenses and solution,
   158–159, 240
cookware, 32–33
coolers and freezer packs,
   176–177, 238
cosmetics, 144, 239. See
   also health and beauty
cotton squares, 146–147,
   239
cotton swabs, 148, 239
crafts, arts and, 70–71,
   236
cutting boards, 36

D

decorations. *See* special occasions

dental care. *See* health and beauty

dental floss, 139, 239

deodorants, 141, 239

detox plan, 30-day, 221–232

about: overview of, 221

week one: at home, 222–223

week two: food and drink, 224–225

halfway point check-in, 227

week three: health and beauty, 228–229

week four: on the go, 230–232

diapers, 43–49

Diwali lamps, 210–211

dogs. *See* pets

drinks. *See* food and drink

dry cleaning, 56

E

earphones. *See* headsets

earplugs, 157, 240

Easter baskets, 207

education, reducing pollution with, 14–15

Eid al-Fitr, gift for, 206

electronics and e-waste, 67, 235. *See also* headsets; phone cases

envelopes, mailing, 74

environment

greenwashing and, 12–14

impact of plastic, 11

microplastics in the ocean, 11

exercise

athletic shoes, 182, 241

yoga mats, 184–185, 241

F

feminine care, 151, 240

festivities. *See* special occasions

filters, water, 37, 234

flowers, for decor, 192–193

food and drink. *See also* baby products

about: 30-day detox plan and, 224–225; overview of, 85; resources, 236–238

baby bottles, 43, 234

beer, 95

bread, 100–101

breakfast cereal, 110–111

cheese, 108

coffee, 90

composting scraps, 65, 236

condiments, 109

coolers and freezer packs, 176–177, 238

drinks, 88–89

Eid al-Fitr gift, 206

frozen foods, 105

fruit, 96–97

grocery bags, 20, 233

gum, 117

Hanukkah gelt, 214–215

hotel mini bar, 172

ice cream, 104

meals and snacks on the go, 181

meat and seafood, 99

milk, 94

nut and seed milks, 93

nuts, seeds, and grains, 112

pasta and noodles, 107

school lunches/snacks, 118–119

snacks, 116

straws, 123, 238

takeout containers, 120

tea, 91

Thanksgiving feast, 212–213

trail mix and snack bars, 113–115

travel drinks, 179

trick or treats, 209

utensils, 121, 237

vegetables, 98

water bottles, 19, 233

water filters, 37, 234

yogurt, 102–103

food storage, 39

food wraps, wax, 41–42

freezer packs, 176, 238

frozen foods, 105

fruit, 96–97

furoshiki, 199

G

games and toys, 69, 235–236

garbage. *See* waste disposal

gardening pots, 81, 236

gifts

about: resources, 242

Easter baskets, 207

for Eid al-Fitr, 206

gift bags, 202

ideas for, 197

Valentines (homemade bath salts gift), 204–205

wrap and ribbon for, 199

glue, 79

grains, nuts, and seeds, 112

greenwashing, 12–14

greeting cards, 190–191, 241

gum, 117

H

hairbrushes and combs, 132, 238

hair care. *See* health and beauty
Halloween costumes, 209
handkerchiefs, 150 239
hand sanitizers, 175, 241
Hanukkah gelt, 214–215
headsets, 170, 241
health and beauty
about: 30-day detox plan and, 228–229; overview of products chemicals, and alternatives, 127; resources, 238–240
bandages, 156, 240
combs and hairbrushes, 132, 238
contact lenses and solution, 158–159, 240
cosmetics, 144, 239
cotton squares, 146–147, 239
cotton swabs, 148, 239
dental floss, 139, 239
deodorants, 141, 239
earplugs, 157, 240
feminine care 151, 240
hair color, 135
hair gel and spray, 133
hair ties, 134
handkerchiefs, 150, 239
homemade bath salts gift, 204–205
insect repellents, 155, 240
makeup removers, 145
moisturizers, 128–129, 238
mouthwash, 140, 239
razors and shaving creams, 142-143, 239
shampoos and conditioners, 131, 238
soaps, 130, 238
sunscreens, 153, 240
toilet paper, 149, 239
toothbrushes, 137, 239
toothpaste, 138, 239

travel toiletries, 171
high-density polyethylene (HDPE), 16, 74, 110
history of plastic, 9–10
holidays. *See* special occasions
home entertainment, 66, 235
hotel key cards, 174, 240
hotel mini bar, 172
household suggestions. *See also* baby products; bed and bath; cleaning solutions and supplies; clothing; food and drink; kids' stuff; kitchen; office and shipping supplies; pets
about: 30-day detox plan and, 222–223; overview of, 25
air fresheners, 59
electronics, 67, 235
gardening pots, 81, 236
home entertainment, 66, 235

I
ice cream, 104
insect repellents, 155, 240
invitations, party, 190-191, 241

K
key cards, hotel, 174, 240
kids' stuff. *See also* baby products
about: resources, 234
arts and crafts, 70–71, 236
tableware and cups, 45
toys and games, 69 235–236
kitchen. *See also* cleaning solutions and supplies; food and drink

about: resources, 234
appliances, 31
bags for groceries, etc., 20, 233
composting scraps, 65, 236
cookware, 32–33
cutting boards, 36
food storage and wax food wraps, 39, 41–42
kids' tableware and cups, 45
napkins and towels, 38
table linens, 196, 242
utensils, 35, 237
water filters, 37

L
lamps, Diwali, 210–211
laundry, 29, 30, 54–55
legislative actions, 15
lighters, 183, 241
linens, bed and bath, 29
linens, table, 196, 242
low-density polyethylene (LDPE), 17, 74, 95, 98
Lunar New Year celebration, 203

M
mailing envelopes, 74
makeup removers, 145. *See also* health and beauty
mattresses, 26
meals. *See* food and drink
meat and seafood, 99
microplastics
cutting boards and, 36
glitter and, 219
negative impacts of, 11
pervasiveness of, 11
washing clothes and, 29, 30
milk, 94
milks, nut and seed, 93

mixed (other) plastic, 17, 66
moisturizers, 128–129, 238
mouthwash, 140, 239

N

napkins and towels, 38
New Year's Eve decorations,
    219. *See also* Lunar New
    Year celebration
noodles and pasta, 107
nut and seed milks, 93
nuts, seeds, and grains, 112
nylon, 29, 35, 48, 91, 137,
    138, 167

O

office and shipping
    supplies
    business cards, 165
    electronics, 67, 235
        (*See also* home
        entertainment)
    glue, 79
    mailing envelopes, 74
    packing materials, 73,
        236
    pens, 76–77, 236
    phone cases, 166, 240
    plates and bowls, 178,
        238
    printer cartridges, 75,
        236
    tape, 78
on the go (travel, work, and
    exercise), 161–184
    about: 30-day detox
        plan and, 230–232;
        overview of plastic
        and disposability, 163;
        resources, 240–242
    athletic shoes, 182, 241
    business cards, 165
    coolers and freezer
        packs, 176–177, 238
    hand sanitizers, 175, 241

headsets, 170, 241
hotel key cards, 174, 240
hotel mini bar, 172
lighters, 183, 241
phone cases, 166, 240
plates and bowls, 178,
    238
receipts and tickets, 164,
    240
suitcases, 167, 241
toiletries for, 171
travel and eco-friendly
    locations, 169, 240
travel drinks, 179
yoga mats, 184–185, 241
ornaments, Christmas,
    216–217

P

packing materials, 73, 236
paper, greenwashing of,
    13
parties. *See* special
    occasions
pasta and noodles, 107
pens, 76–77, 236
pets
    about: resources, 235
    accessories, 53
    food, 51
    waste (cat and dog), 52
phone cases, 166, 240
phthalates, 27, 31, 47, 53, 59,
    70, 91, 127, 184
plastic
    benefits of, 10–11
    detox plan (*See* detox
        plan, 30-day)
    detrimental impact of, 11
    environmental damage, 11
    the good, bad, and ugly
        of, 10–11
    greenwashing of, 12–14
    history of, 9–10
    paper vs., 13

from plant cellulose, 9–10
production statistics, 10
relationship with, 7–8
types of, abbreviations,
    uses, and recyclability,
    16–17, 167, 219
ubiquity of, 7, 9
plastic pollution, reducing
    education for, 14–15
    legislative actions, 15
    refuse, reduce, reuse, 15
    resources, 233–242
    solutions, 14–15 (*See also*
        specific solutions)
    water bottles, 19, 233
plates and bowls, 178, 238
Polyethylene terephthalate
    (PET or PETE), uses
    and recyclability, 16
polypropylene (PP), 17, 47,
    48, 91, 102, 167
polystyrene (PS), 17, 69, 73,
    76, 99
Poly-T, 39
polytetrafluoroethylene
    (PTFE), 32
polyurethane (PU), 26, 48,
    60, 63, 156
polyvinyl chloride (PVC,
    Vinyl), 17, 27, 46, 51, 53,
    156, 174, 184, 196, 197,
    216
pots and pans, 32
pots, gardening, 81, 236
printer cartridges, 75, 236

R

razors and shaving creams,
    142–143, 239
receipts and tickets, 164,
    240
recycling
    greenwashing and, 12
    limitations and cost, 12
    reality of, 12